AF894629

indayi
edition

Cancer is preventable – cancer is vincible

A book for the whole family, for physicians, healers, sick and healthy.

Visit us at:

www.indayi.de

indayi edition

Bibliographic information of the German National Library:
The German National Library lists this publication in the German National Bibliography; detailed bibliographic data are available on the Internet at
http://dnb.d-nb.de.

1st edition June 2021

© indayi edition, Darmstadt

All rights reserved. The work may be reproduced - even in part - only with the permission of the publisher.

Image credits: Moringa amazingwellnessmag.com, Oil bottle Pixelio Uwe Wagschal, Palm oil oneVillage Initiative, via Wikimedia Commons, Onion Amada44, via Wikimedia Commons, Ginger Mgmoscatello, via Wikimedia Commons, Garlic Dubravko Sorić Sora, via Wikimedia Commons, Banana collection TimothyPilgrim via wikimedia commons, Raspberry Theo Crazzolara via wikimedia commons, Safou http://www.rohkostwiki.de/wiki/Safu, Graviola Muhammad Mahdi Karim via Wikimedia Commons, Citrus http://www.besserhaushalten.de/rezepte-kochen/kochtipps/vitaminkick-durch-zitrusfruechte.html, Mango http://www.afribiz.info/wp-content/uploads/2012/01/rsz_wild-mango_kuini_asit_ftg-wikimedia-1.jpg, bitacola http://www.stylishranchgirl.com/wp-content/uploads/2014/09/kola-nut.jpg, guava https://commons.wikimedia.org/wiki/File:Psidium_guajava_fruit.jpg, baobab Lix via Wikimedia Commons, habanero http://www.habanerosocial.com/wp-content/uploads/2013/12/habanero-peppers-1.jpg, yams http://www.fraichacademy.fr/ligname/, cassava Anneli Salo via Wikimedia Commons, coconut and coconut oil http://www.jenny.gr/h-epidrash-tou-coconut-oil-sto-alzheimer/, shea butter https://simplesoaparie.files.wordpress.com/2015/07/shea-butter-in-bowl.jpg, fried plantain Dmitri via Wikimedia Commons

Cover design, typesetting and editing: Birgit Pretzsch
Translation: Adrian Burger
Edit translation: Janina Jura

ISBN: 978-3-947003-62-4

The ultimate
Anti-
CANCE
R
book

Our diet –
friend and foe

Cancer cell feeders

Cancer cell killers

Cancer cell preventers

with new insights and top tips, that really help

African inspired – scientifically profound

by Dantse Dantse

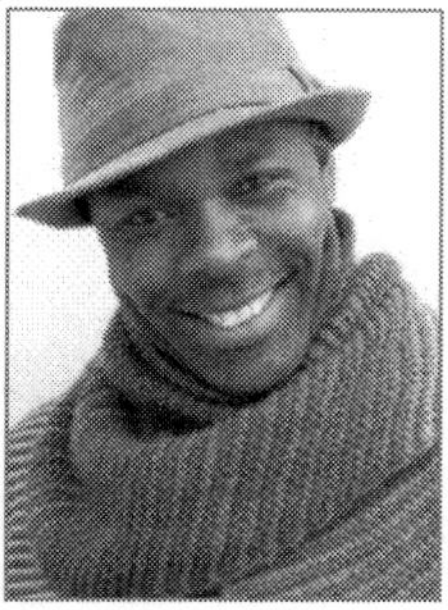

About the author

Dantse Dantse was born in Cameroon, studied in Germany and has lived in Darmstadt for over 25 years. He is the father of five children, a kind of person usually called a "Connoisseur of the art of living". Unconventional, free in his person and in his way of thinking, independent of the established, but which he fully respects.

As a child, he lived with a total of 25 children. His father had three officially married wives at the same time, all living together in one facility. Values such as giving, sharing, feelings, love, jealousy, patience, sympathizing with others and many more have a different emphasis than in a so-called "normal" family. These childhood experiences, his African roots, the European cultural influence on him and his years of coaching experience let him see things differently, act differently and be different, which has something refreshing.

As the first African to found a book publishing house in Germany, indayi edition, and as an unconventional author, he likes to write and publish books that reflect his intercultural experiences, books about values and about topics that society does not like to address and prefers to sweep under the carpet, but which affect millions of people, such as homosexuality in Africa, female circumcision, sexuality, organ trafficking, racism, mental disorders, sexual abuse, and so on. He writes and publishes books that aim to explain, change and improve things - be it his guidebooks, non-fiction books, novels, children's books or political blog comments.

Inspired by his insights and knowledge from Africa, which he learned in many teachings, from his own extreme experiences and experiments - such as the excessive intake of sugar to study the effect on the psyche - from scientific studies and research and from experiences of other parts of the world, he is very successfully helping women, men and children through his coaching in the areas of nutrition, health, career, stress, burnout, spirituality, body, family and love. With Dantse Dantse you master your life!

His distinctive writing style, influenced by his African and French mother tongues, is his distinguishing feature and has been preserved in the text and only carefully edited.

DantseLOGIC™
Master Your Life

DantseLOGIC™
Master Your Relationship

DantseLOGIC™
Master Your Family

DantseLOGIC™
Master Your Weight

DantseLOGIC™
Master Your Health

DantseLOGIC™
Master Your Career

DantseLOGIC™
Master Your Communication

DantseLOGIC™
Master Your Crisis

DantseLOGIC™
Master Your Stress

DantseLOGIC™
Master Your Femininity

DantseLOGIC™
Master Your Masculinity

All brands by

DANTSE™
Meistere dein Leben

Coaching that works like magic - that is the motto of the

DantseLOGIC™
Master Your Life

-DantseLOGIC. Logic that works wonders.

-DantseLOGIC. Logic that moves.

-DantseLOGIC. Logic that makes you happy.

-DantseLOGIC. The power to succeed.

-DantseLOGIC. Heals. Works. Guaranteed.

Explanation: Why should you read this book?

In just two weeks of dietary change, from the Western diet to the African diet, subjects in a scientific study of Americans showed first signs of a reduction in risk of developing colon cancer.

How is that possible in just two weeks?

In this study, as in numerous before and after it, it is shown that food plays an important role in the development or control of cancer.

Many of the things you will read about in this book are known to the pharmaceutical industry, because they use them to produce medicines. It knows very well that some of the African foods can work miracles. All these African foods have been deeply researched and their healing power is known and documented. But people only talk about them and spread the knowledge when they have created a medicine from them and patented it. Only when one can generate money with it, the healing power of the substances is made public. Examples are yam or ginger and their effect against cancer. Only when capsules and teas were made from them, the effect of these plants was suddenly also known to be anticarcinogenic, although many natural physicians in Cameroon and in many other countries have been using the healing substances of these roots since time immemorial.

When I talked to people in Germany 20 years ago about the healing power of ginger, I was laughed at. But today ginger products are big business and suddenly everyone is talking about it. It is the same with many other foods that help us and can cure many diseases, but they are unknown to the masses.

That's why I decided to write a book about this ugly disease, cancer, in which I share these insights and secrets that the pharmaceutical industry has acquired with people, some of which come from Africa. It is no coincidence that there are continents like Africa where cancer is virtually unknown in certain areas. This has to do with nutrition, as the following study shows.

Table of contents

Study: African diet showed cancer risk reduction in just two weeks

In just two weeks of dietary changes from a Western to an African diet, African-Americans showed early signs of a reduced risk of developing colorectal cancer, according to a scientific study. Colorectal cancer is one of the most common types of cancer in Western countries and the second most deadly type.

A study about the connection between Western dietary patterns and cancer was conducted with African-Americans and Africans. African-Americans have many times higher rates of colorectal cancer than Africans from rural southern Africa. This difference was largely explained by differences in diet, according to the study. Particularly with high-risk individuals, a high-fiber diet can have an extremely positive effect on colorectal cancer risk. People from both groups were used for the study. The African-Americans, with their Western-oriented diet (many animal proteins and animal fat) and the Africans, with their high-fiber diet.

American and British scientists began studying the diet of 20 African-Americans and 20 Africans in the KwaZulu-Natal province of South Africa. They found that African-Americans ate two to three times more fat and animal protein than Africans. In addition, they ate much less fiber than people in Africa.

The researchers then analyzed the gut flora of the two groups. They found that the American and African diets were associated with very different populations of gut bacteria. The Africans had more bacteria that proliferate through carbohydrate fermentation and others that produce butyric acid. The Americans had more bacteria that break down bile acids. Colonoscopy showed the presence of polyps, which can sometimes turn into tumors, in 9 Americans. These polyps were not present in any African.

The scientists then asked the two groups to switch their diet for two weeks. Instead of their normal meals, rich in fiber, the Africans ate a diet high in fat, chips, cake, burgers and food high in animal protein. African-Americans have been eating a low-fat diet rich in fiber, consisting of legumes, vegetables, and fruits.

After two weeks, the teams from the University of Pittsburgh and the Imperial College of London analyzed the results. They found that the African-Americans had significantly less inflammations of the colon and that cancer biomarkers were decreased. That was not the case for the Africans. They appeared to have signs of increased cancer risk (increase in inflammations). "We were impressed by the magnitude of the changes. We thought we would find a few changes here and there, but what we found was completely unexpected," said Stephen O'Keefe, the study's principal investigator. **"The results suggest that it's never too late to reduce the risk of colorectal cancer,"** he added.

The changes in cancer risk coincided with dramatic changes in the gut bacteria population. With the high-fiber diet, gut bacteria produce more butyric acid, while the Western diet leads to increased production of bile acids, which can increase cancer risk. Many other studies have shown that a diet rich in fiber reduces the risk of developing colorectal cancer, although it has not yet been possible to explain exactly how the mechanism works.

This study suggests that diet may have an effect on cancer risk, via changes in gut flora and substances released in the bowel.

Study: African diet showed cancer risk reduction in just two weeks

Source: http://www.nature.com/articles/ncomms7342 (Published April 2015)

Preface part 1: A wrong, bad and unhealthy diet causes cancer

It is estimated that dietary influences are partly responsible for one third of all cases of cancer in industrialized countries. In the Western world, cancer is a fear-inducing disease, being the second leading cause of death after cardiovascular disease. But it wasn't always this way. Cancer used to be a rare disease that affected only few people. 100 years ago, very few people died of cancer.

In Germany, almost 500,000 people are diagnosed with cancer every year, and more than half of them, around 224,000 people, die. The most common type of cancer in men is prostate cancer, in women breast cancer and in children it is leukemia. Overall, it can be said that cancer is a disease of the so-called affluent nations. According to studies, 40% of new cases occurred in countries with a very high level of development in 2008, although they make up only 15% of the world's population. But cancer is also on the rise in emerging and developing countries, because many people there have abandoned their old lifestyles and eating habits to adopt those of the so-called Western nations.

4 years ago, when I decided to write the book "Cancerous Generations", I talked to many medical doctors from both directions (conventional and natural medicine) in Cameroon who were taking care of cancer patients. I found that many of the patients they treated were people who had reached a certain standard of living. Many of these people frequently shopped at the supermarket and excessively ate canned foods from Europe.

Preface part 1:
A wrong, bad and unhealthy diet causes cancer

Breakfast now included over-sugared Nestlé cans of condensed milk, or powdered milk full of chemicals, sausages, imported chicken that contained so much hormones that men developed breasts after only a few months, etc. This trend was even clearer recognizable among children. More and more African children are getting cancer since many ingredients in children's food and drinks come from China. Some sodas in Cameroon are virtually poison. This colored water contains up to 90% artificial sugar and the children love it. It was clear to experts - whether they were naturopaths or conventional doctors - that the changes in eating habits in Cameroon were promoting the development of cancer. This was consistent with the trend of worldwide scientific evidence. These were further strong indications that poor diet increases the risk of cancer.

Cancer can be preventable to some extent. Proper diet and a healthy lifestyle can prevent many cases of cancer, poor diet and unhealthy lifestyle can spread it. Proper nutrition does not only mean eating healthy food or eating organic products. Proper nutrition also means eating the right foods. Likewise, a wrong nutrition means eating the wrong foods or avoiding certain foods. The influence of nutrition on the development of cancer thus lies mainly in its potential to promote cancer through wrong food choices.

I spent a lot of my free time with naturopaths and saw them helping and explaining to people how valuable Cameroonian foods are, what they can fight, eliminate and cure, and equally why the Western diet stimulates cancer. Which foods and substances in the diet cause cancer to develop or increase the risk? I have compiled certain facts from many studies, from findings in Africa and from my coaching, which I show in this book.

Preface part 2: We do not surrender to cancer

A specific African diet can successfully curb cancer. Diet can probably fight cancer successfully.

A French doctor said to my father, "The active agents of many drugs that we have patented here in Europe come from African plants and foods. African foods are a holistic pharmacy, and we make billions with it."

If the drugs would not generate a lot of money and profit, we could cure many chronic diseases today with the help of nature. But our misfortune is that so much money is made with the drugs. A plant is only valuable when the pharmaceutical industry has patented its active agent and can sell it. Large parts of what we swallow from the pharmacy to be healthy come from nature. The best friends of natural remedies are not only the naturopaths. Conventional medicine also makes use of a large extent of findings from nature and of what foods are and what they can do.

Inspired by my insights and knowledge from Africa, learned from many teachings, my own experiences and experiments, analysis of scientific studies and research and experiences from other parts of the world, I help women, men and children to become healthier through my coaching as a nutritionist. To bring these great insights to more people and help more people, I decided to write this book series.

You'll generally be amazed at how many of your ailments are eliminated if you change your diet, how it makes you healthy and you'll be amazed at how much weight you lose in the process, how much muscle you build up and how much more vital and happy you are. It's almost magical.

Many foods have preventive and especially lasting effect against cancer. It is important to eat different foods at the same time and adopt a healthy diet as the basic basis of the eating habit.

Even if you just follow a part of the advice in this book, you will see how quickly you feel better. You will be pleased to find that many of your ailments disappear quickly. I am very sure of this! If not, contact me and together we will see why it is not working.

In this book, you will receive general advice on how to strengthen, protect, or regain your health holistically with natural foods and how to prevent cancer from now on or, if you suffer from cancer, how to use food to curb or even stop its spread.

This book in no way replaces medical consultations or visits to the doctor, but it will help you to strengthen your health, prevent diseases and support medical therapy. It makes you feel good again, strengthens your self-confidence and promotes a better contact with yourself. Because nature is you and you are nature. To deal with natural foods and other natural remedies is to understand yourself better. Those who know and understand themselves well live healthier, happier and more peaceful lives, so says an African proverb.

I expand your knowledge and enrich you with a lot of new information and exclusive knowledge about new substances and foods, as you will rarely read in a book. This is only possible because I bring a lot from Africa with me, new foods with amazing healing powers that are known to some researchers and science, but not yet to ordinary people.

This book is written in a simple way and easy to understand for everyone; here you will find a lot of useful and detailed information gathered in one place:

- **A list of all vitamins and minerals: in which foods they are found, their anti-cancer function, what causes a deficiency**
- **A list of anti-cancer vitamins and minerals**
- **A list of toxins and chemicals in foods that cause cancer and countermeasures**
- **Alkaline, bitter, acidic foods and how they work against cancer**
- **All about antioxidants, what foods they are found in and how they kill cancer cells**
- **A list of some tropical foods with strong anti-cancer healing power**
- **A list of African miracle carbohydrates, most effective anti-cancer fighters**
- **A detailed listing of many anti-cancer foods by food type: anti-cancer fruits, anti-cancer nuts, anti-cancer vegetables, anti-cancer fats and much more.**
- **Explanation why vegetable oil is indispensable in the fight against cancer**
- **How to get a healthy intestinal flora and why this is the basis of the successful fight against cancer**
- **How the sun prevents cancer and inhibits cancer cells**
- **Natural antibiotics**

- **African-inspired cooking recipes for a complete week that effectively prevent cancer and prevent the development of cancer cells**
- **And much more**

The book is intentionally free of complicated jargon and technical definitions that no one really understands anyway, so that you can act directly, without much thought, and understand what is good for you.

A starter book for every woman and man to keep you looking for yourself and understand how much of which foods you eat determines your health.

This blend of science, my holistic coaching and my knowledge from Africa makes this book a wealth of knowledge for a healthy life and is good for people dealing with cancer.

ATTENTION:

The health and medical information provided for you in this book and in all my books is not a substitute for medical advice or treatment.

Part 1

How diet causes cancer:

CANCER

likes wheat
loves sugar
and smooches milk
How diet causes cancer

Carcinogenic toxicants in food
and baby food

A. HOW DIET MAKES US SICK AND WHITE FLOUR MAKES US STUPID

Introduction

For years I have been studying the connection of disease and food. Inspired by my findings and knowledge from Africa, which I have learned in many teachings, from my own experiences and experiments, from scientific studies and research and from experiences from other parts of the world, I decided to write this book to show as many people as possible that many ailments result directly from our poor diet.

This book does not replace medical consultations and doctor's visits at all, but it helps you to understand better, to prevent diseases, and to support medical therapies. It makes you feel good about yourself again and strengthens your self-confidence and promotes a better contact with yourself. Because nature is you and you are nature. One who knows oneself well and understands oneself well, lives healthier, happier and more peaceful, so says an African proverb.

In modern conventional medicine and in the medical community, diseases, their causes and their treatment are often explained and treated differently than one does from a holistic point of view. The medical community tries to understand diseases locally. From a holistic and natural point of view, one looks at the entire organism and rarely at individual symptoms. While, for example, conventional medicine wants to cure cancer only with drugs (which bring even more side effects), natural medicine aims to bring the whole organism back into its healthy balance and combines drugs with the whole life situation of the sick person so that conventional medicine works successfully. This is also my approach. A human being cannot be separated, not into its individual parts, not from the society it lives in, not from its family, not from its profession, not from its sexuality, not from nature, because it is a part of it and that means it cannot be separated from where it lives, what it thinks, eats, drinks and breathes. That is why many natural methods have sometimes worked for a long time, although conventional medicine is only now finding out certain connections. In the case of cancer it is important to restore the whole balance as well.

I expand your knowledge and enrich you with a lot of new information and exclusive knowledge about substances and foods, as rarely before.

This book is written in a simple way and easy to understand for everyone; here you will find a lot of useful and detailed information gathered in one place:

- Why dairy products, sugar and wheat are enemies of our health
- Which beverages harm our body
- Vitamins and minerals: what effects deficiencies have
- Additives (preservatives, colorants, etc.) in food, sorted by where they are found and what they cause
- Toxins and chemicals in food and countermeasures
- Free radicals

- A list of which foods promote cancer
- A list of which foods promote which diseases

  And much more

The book is intentionally free of complicated technical terms and technical definitions that no one really understands anyway, so that you can act directly, without much thought and understand what is harming you. A handbook for every woman and man, so that you continue to search and understand how big of an impact of which food you eat has on your health.

This blend of science, my holistic coaching and knowledge from Africa makes this book a wealth of knowledge for a healthy life and is good for people dealing with cancer.

Let's start first with the book, "This is how diet makes us sick and white flour makes us stupid", which I have integrated into this book, because it already contains a lot of useful information about foods that promote or increase cancer.

Part B is even more specific about cancer:

- What cancer is
- What environment favors the development of cancer
- Which foods promote cancer
- An entire list of carcinogenic chemicals and toxins in foods, depending on the type of food
- A list of carcinogens in baby foods
- And much more

A1 General connections between disease and nutrition: What is disease and why do we get sick?

With technical and industrial development, many new diseases have emerged and some old diseases have become more aggressive and dangerous. On the one hand, many diseases can be cured today, on the other hand, people have "invented" even more diseases. We live unhealthier today than the people before us.

Why do we get sick? Illness is defined as a disturbance of physical and mental functions. The functions of life also include behavior and emotions. This means that we get sick when something has thrown our body out of balance. The disease is therefore a reaction, often a defense of the body against a foreign "attack".

The disease usually manifests itself through external symptoms. These symptoms are very important because they make it clear to us that something is wrong and that something should be done to regain physical balance. They are aids.

Many diseases can be psychological or physical and are caused by stress, negative thoughts, fear, poor lifestyle, accidents, lack of exercise, side effects of medications, viruses and bacteria, environmental toxins, heavy physical exertion and poor nutrition. It is nutrition, along with mental attitude that perhaps plays the greatest role in the onset, development and elimination of disease.

With nutrition, we can fight many diseases in advance, before they occur, or quickly eliminate them if we do get sick. This also means that with the wrong diet and bad food we can also promote diseases.

A2 The most common causes of disease are found in poor nutrition

Many studies show that people in industrialized countries eat poorly. These studies show that more than half of the adults in Germany are overweight. 2/3 of men and 51% of women put too many kilos on the scales.

The German diet is unhealthy, animal fats have pushed the healthy vegetable fat out of the market. People eat too sweet, too acidic, too many ready meals, too many artificial additives and too many dairy products. Ready meals and processed foods contain vast amounts of chemicals that make burning fat impossible. The higher the amount of fat and sugar, the greater the amount of calories.

In addition, their drinking habits are often extremely unhealthy: artificially produced beverages, doped up with chemicals and preservatives (e.g. soft drinks), lots of alcohol, sometimes still in the fatal combination with artificial sweeteners (e.g. alcopops). At the same time, Germans do very little exercise. People hardly ever cook and if they do, it is often of inferior quality! The consequence is obesity. Obesity significantly increases the risk of cancer and allows the cancer to spread more and faster.

In the other volumes of this series, you will learn that by eating the right foods, you can not only stay healthy, but also reach and maintain your desired weight without "cruel" effort, abandonment and depression. With these tips, you will eat a filling and varied diet and you will not only be guaranteed to lose weight, but also build muscle, improve cellulite and orange peel skin and get smoother and firmer skin. You will also note that you are more active and less tired, your concentration will increase, you will feel younger and your overall quality of life will improve. You'll simply notice that you're happier and more in tune with your body. But that's not all! My tips and tricks will also stimulate desire and passion during sex in the long run!

In this volume, however, we first look at which foods make us sick.

The big danger with food is not just the food itself, but the added chemicals (additives, fertilizers, pesticides, etc.) and the way the agricultural products are processed.

Many sources of disease are found in modern agriculture, animal breeding and factory farming, and the food processing industry.

Humans poison themselves in several ways:

- Directly through the chemicals in the agricultural products
- Through the chemicals and substances used to process these products into various food products
- Through meat of animals fed with the agricultural products
- Through meat of animals raised with chemicals (such as hormones) and drugs
- Through meat of animals processed with additives and other chemicals
- Through artificially produced food
- Through genetically modified food
- In addition to this, poisoning through chemicals in the beverage industry
- Through interaction of individual substances in one or more products simultaneousl

A3 Intestinal disorders and an unhealthy intestinal flora prevent weight loss and cause diseases

Your health lies in your intestines and whether you lose weight or not is often decided right there. A sick intestine means not only little and insufficient protection against attacks from the outside (such as from environmental toxins), fast and frequent infections because of a weak immune system (a large part - over 80% - of our immune system lies in our intestine), but also sluggish fat loss, because of sluggish digestive processes.

The intestinal flora is disturbed or even destroyed by poor nutrition, high alcohol consumption, some medications (radiation or chemotherapy, antibiotics, cortisone) and environmental toxins.

The intestinal flora is mainly located in the large intestine, where more than 400 different species of bacteria are found, such as lactic acid bacteria or coli bacteria; these are called intestinal bacteria.

Studies have shown that overweight people have an unhealthier intestinal flora than normal weight people and this prevents digestion from proceeding normally. It was found that overweight women did not lose weight despite dieting, but once they had "cleaned up" their flora, for example with a probiotic, they lost twice as much weight without dieting as overweight women who dieted.

The first typical symptoms of a sick intestine may be:

- Flatulence
- A weak immune system,
- Gas in the stomach

- Hemorrhoids
- Long-lasting fatigue and listlessness
- Bad breath
- Sudden diarrhea, often watery
- Poor skin appearance
- Hiccup
- Heartburn
- Constant stomach and abdominal pain
- Constant constipation, slow digestion
- Intolerances
- Feeling of fullness that stays for a long time, often after eating, even though you haven't eaten much at all

A3.1 Sick intestinal flora, health and cancer

Healers in Africa see a clear connection between a disturbed intestinal flora and a variety of diseases. The processes in the gut even influence our mood and vice versa (the so-called "gut feeling" was not invented, it is reality. My naturopathic teacher called it the "third eye" in us).

An imbalance in the natural composition of the different types of bacteria destabilizes the intestinal flora and we become sick.

Each cell is only as healthy as the quality of the nutrients (free of toxins) that nourish it. Nutrients are processed in the intestine by the "good" intestinal bacteria and absorbed by the healthy intestinal mucosa. The separation of nutrients and toxins begins in the intestines. A sick intestine, on the other hand, produces toxins or cannot stop toxins, it can no longer guarantee that healthy nutrients, free of toxins, reach the cells. Thus, the cells are supplied with toxins, which permanently disrupt the digestive and metabolic processes. Without healthy cells, there is no health. Now we understand why the origin of our health lies in intestinal health.

The modern way of eating makes the intestine susceptible to diseases: Too many foods rich in flour, milk and sugar with many chemicals (additives). The modern and western civilization diseases lurk in the intestine. The industrial diet style is enemy of the intestinal flora. Many diseases emerge because the intestinal flora is sick and disturbed.

The following diseases can be caused by a diseased intestinal flora:

- Allergies
- Autoimmune diseases, such as neurodermatitis
- Anemia
- Chronic fatigue
- Chronic inflammation
- Diabetes
- Gastroenteritis
- Mental illnesses such as depression, eating disorders, confusion, anxiety, stress
- Diarrhea

- Skin diseases
- Immunodeficiency
- Susceptibility to infection
- Cancer (pancreatic cancer, colon cancer)
- Liver damage due to intestinal toxins
- Stomach/intestinal pain, intestinal cramps, stomach ulcers
- Intestinal inflammation
- Fatigue and lack of concentration as consequences of liver damage due to intestinal toxins
- Constant migraines and headaches
- Food intolerances
- Vitamin and mineral deficiencies, especially iron, due to poor nutrient intake
- Fungal infections
- Vaginal yeast infection
- Fungal infections of the glans
- Urinary tract infections
- Inflammation oft he bladder especially after sex
- Pain during or after sex

Especially people who have undergone antibiotic therapy have a sick intestinal flora afterwards, because antibiotics destroy the intestinal flora.

Nitrosamines can also upset the intestinal flora: These substances damage the intestinal wall and can thus cause tumors. If there is a lot of nitrite (e.g. in cured foods) but little or no vitamin C in the food, nitrosamines can develop. Nitrosamines also enter our bodies directly from agriculture, because nitrate is widely used as fertilizer. When heating food that has been in contact with this fertilizer, nitrate turns into nitrite. And that's how quickly you can "go bad" with supposedly healthy vegetables.

A4 What foods are harmful to health?

A4.1 Milk and dairy products: A danger to health

If your life were as bitter as mine, and you had to witness this massacre of innocent children by a totally inappropriate diet day by day, I believe you would feel exactly as I do: This misguided propaganda about infant nutrition should rather be considered as the murder of children. Anyone who, through ignorance or even recklessness, causes a baby to be fed unsuitable food can be found guilty of the baby's death. - Dr. Cicely Williams, Milk and Murder, 1939. She was a prominent pediatrician and gave this speech in Singapore in 1939. (http://www.zentrum-der-gesundheit.de/babynahrung.html)

The assumption that milk is very rich in calcium and therefore healthy is deceptive, because cow's milk production is extremely unhealthy. What the cows eat to produce that much milk makes the milk a health risk.

Consuming a lot of dairy products causes many problems in our body and in our psyche. Milk contributes to the fact that our body is overacidified and thus many bacteria have the opportunity to emerge, multiply and feel right at home.

For example, studies have shown that Asians (Chinese and Japanese) were hardly aware of the so-called diseases of civilization until they began to drink milk on a large scale, consume dairy products and use them in cooking.

In Cameroon, there used to be no animal husbandry for milk at all, as it has been known for thousands of years that animal milk is not meant for humans, and even less so when they are already adults. But even in Cameroon, it was quickly observed that people who adopted the Western dietary method with lots of milk and dairy products and ready meals also suffered more frequently from these diseases of civilization. Almost all ready meals from the supermarket are prepared with milk.

Dairy products promote the development of cancer

In my book "Cancerous Generation", I wrote a lot about this in connection with cancer. Here is an excerpt;

"...As with pills, chemotherapy, radiotherapy and some medications, when it comes to dairy products, opinions vary widely and are highly controversial, even among scientists. Some think that because of the high calcium content and the almost ideal ratio of proteins, fats and carbohydrates in milk, milk and milk derivatives are excellent foods. But many studies warn that milk and dairy products can also cause cancer. Milk contains high levels of estrogen and progesterone, which can significantly increase breast, ovarian and uterine cancer risk. Dairy cows' feed has very little to do with greens, and all the more to do with concentrated feed, which is still diligently laced with chemicals and toxins (pesticides, herbicides, fungicides, drugs, etc.), critics say. Their criticism is fueled by the increasing prevalence of lactose intolerance in the population. Cow's milk is also healthy for calves only during the time when they cannot yet eat grass. Nature did not intend for humans to still drink milk in adulthood, they stress.

Some studies demonstrated an increased risk of cancer from milk, others did not come to this conclusion. As always, opponents and supporters accuse each other of being conspiracy theorists, scaremongers or money sharks, scientists in the pay of business and capital.

It is clear that milk and dairy products are the staple foods in Western countries. Most dishes, pastries, cakes, chocolate, sweets, contain more or less something that is made of milk. That is why milk is essential for the economy and food industry and in the end we consumers cannot know exactly what is true and what is not. Also reports in the media can be tendentious because of this.

Well, what does a serious scientific study from Harvard University have to say about this?

In the spirit of this book, I would like to present facts and information from my research that should lead consumers to broaden their view of milk and better assess risks.

Even if it is assumed that milk would be healthy, the question is whether the industrially processed cow's milk is also still valuable? In order for the milk to remain durable, it is heated, filtered and processed (pasteurized, homogenized, etc.). The ingredients of the milk are thus altered and lose their effectiveness. The new milk no longer has anything to do with the natural milk. For example, the good fat is so finely filtered by this industrial process that it is no longer as good for the human body as the original fat.

A Harvard University study finds a link between cancer and pasteurized (industrial) milk-

A group of scientists, led by Doctor Ganmaa Davaasambuu, sees a link between pasteurized milk and cases of cancer (breast cancer, prostate cancer, ovarian cancer), according to a study. Industrially processed milk in the USA was examined. Natural milk from Mongolia served as a comparative value. In particular, hormone-dependent types of cancer such as breast or prostate cancer (maybe my mother was right after all when she said that milk can cause problems in the genital area of men?) are said to be favored by industrial milk. In this study, industrial milk was found to contain 33 times more estrogen than Mongolia's natural milk. Doctor Davaasambuu told the Harvard Gazette: "The milk we drink today may have nothing to do with nature's perfect food."

The study suspects the causes in the type of feed and animal husbandry in modern farms. The animals' feed is mixed with hormones and drugs, and these get into the milk. According to the Harvard study, there would be a possible link between the female sex hormones in the milk of pregnant cows and the development of breast ovarian and uterine cancer.

Even earlier cancer studies referred to milk consumption!

An international comparative study confirmed Dr. Davaasambuu's hypothesis that consumption of dairy products increases the likelihood of cancer. The connection between dietary habits and cancer rates in 42 countries was studied. It was found that there was a connection between dairy or cheese consumption and testicular cancer. Cancer rates were highest in countries such as Switzerland, where a lot of cheese is consumed. In countries where dairy products are consumed little or rarely, fewer cases were reported.

A clear link between milk and cancer is also emerging in Japan. The number of cases of prostate cancer and breast cancer has risen sharply with increased milk consumption over the last 50 years.

Breast cancer studies again specifically warned against milk and cheese. Another study confirmed that rats fed with milk were more likely to develop tumors than rats that drank water instead.

On the website of Harvard School of Public Health (http://www.hsph.harvard.edu/nutritionsource/what-should-you-eat/calcium-and-milk/) it is said that "... Calcium is important. But milk isn't the only, or even best, source... While calcium and dairy can lower the risk of osteoporosis and colon cancer, high intake can increase the risk of prostate cancer and possibly ovarian cancer."

A report on milk on the website of Bavarian television also confirms the assumption of a link between cancer and dairy products, although the report is very wary: "When is it healthy? When does it make you sick?.. At the moment, studies suggest that increased milk consumption can reduce the risk of colon cancer. Possibly, however, milk consumption increases the risk of prostate cancer. However, only if a lot of calcium is consumed at the same time and little vitamin D..... In other words, you should never eat more than 1,500 mg of calcium per day and make sure that you get enough vitamin D. For breast cancer, the study situation is not clear.... "

Nitrite compounds: It is known that nitrite is present in many cheeses and other dairy products, which can form nitrosamines in the stomach. Many pharmaceuticals form nitrosamine compounds from nitrite together with other foods as well, which are extremely effective carcinogens.

Aflatoxins B1 - very dangerous carcinogenic substance in milk

Aflatoxins are naturally occurring fungal toxins that were first identified in mold.

There are over 20 naturally occurring aflatoxins, of which aflatoxin B1 is considered the most dangerous for humans. In addition to aflatoxin B1, the toxins B2, G1 and G2 and the derivatives M1 and M2, which occur in milk, are of particular importance.

"Aflatoxins have an acute hepatotoxic effect (liver dystrophy) at concentrations around 10 µg/kg body weight, but are carcinogenic to mammals, birds, and fish even at lower concentrations and especially with repeated ingestion. The lethal dose of aflatoxin B1 in adults is 1 to 10 mg/kg body weight when ingested orally. In animal studies with rats (lethal dose 7.2 mg/kg body weight), the carcinogenicity of a daily dose of 10 µg/kg body weight was clearly demonstrated. Aflatoxin B1 is thus one of the most potent carcinogenic compounds of all." (Wikipedia)

Because of the dangerous effects of aflatoxins, limit values (maximum levels) have been set in many countries around the world and also within the European Union.

Aflatoxins are heat-stable and are destroyed only to a small extent during cooking or baking. They can be ingested with food or contaminated air.

If agricultural products containing aflatoxins are fed as animal feed, the aflatoxins can pass into foodstuffs such as milk.

Dioxins and the dioxin-like polychlorinated biphenyls (PCBs)

These chlorine-containing substances are found in milk and milk derivatives and are very toxic, some are even carcinogenic. Since dioxins and PCBs love fat, the risk for humans to ingest these substances increases with the fat content of the food. Dioxins and PCBs are very durable substances. They hardly break down once they are stored in fatty tissue. The older one gets and with continuous intake of the toxins, the higher their content increases in the body and this means a higher probability of cancer.

Milk and osteoporosis and other ailments

In my research, I found old studies showing that milk can lead to osteoporosis. Dr. Ganmaa Davaasambuu comments: "In terms of estrogen exposure for humans, cow's milk worries us the most because it contains a significant amount of female sex hormones."

I know from my own experience what a reduced consumption of milk and dairy products can do and I also know that my clients and many people around me who largely give up dairy products report that they feel better (improvement of body odor and skin, disappearance of migraines, weight loss, especially on the hips and abdomen, disappearance of painful menstruation, strengthening of sexual desire and virility, and much more).

The worldwide continuing increase in the incidence of hormone-controlled types of cancer must compel us to intensively discuss the possible role of endogenous estrogens in the diet as well. As it happens, cow's milk contains a considerable amount of estrogens.

This means that circumstantial evidence is available that should make us humans take a closer look at our attitude toward milk. Maybe the ancient African wisdom is right after all? But I know that a tough controversy will remain about what milk can do and how milk can harm, however. The best thing to do is to go without it for some time to experience the changes in our own bodies and souls."

There is also a possible link between milk and Parkinson's disease or diabetes.

A4.2 White flour causes cancer - white flour makes people depressed

The wheat of modern times has nothing, nothing at all, to do with the healthy wheat of the past. Through breeding and genetic manipulation, many cereal varieties - like wheat - have become a high-performance crop with few nutrients. Wheat today is a cross between different species and contains nearly 50% gluten so that industrial baking processes could be perfected. Just 50 years ago, the amount was only 5% gluten. Gluten gives rise to the elasticity of the dough; without gluten it is practically impossible to produce the baked goods we know.

According to Wikipedia, gluten is a collective term for a mixture of substances made up of proteins found in the seeds of some types of cereals. When water is added to cereal flour, the gluten forms a rubbery and elastic mass from the flour when it rises, namely the dough. The gluten is of central importance for the baking properties of a flour.

Cereals with high gluten content are wheat, spelt, rye, kamut, amelcorn, einkorn. In contrast, millet, corn and rice, quinoa, amaranth and buckwheat are gluten-free. Cereals with little gluten are durum, oat and barley.

The industry also uses gluten as glue and in the same way it glues our body together, hindering the absorption of nutrients. This leads to a lack of nutrients. The consequences for the body are chronic inflammations, which in turn causes chronic diseases such as cancer. Gluten can also cause depression, as researchers at Monash University in Australia have shown. It also accelerates the aging process.

If you have gluten intolerance (celiac disease) or sensitivity, avoid the following grains:

- white flour
- spelt
- rye
- kamut
- einkorn
- quinoa : Quinoa is not directly a grain, but contains prolamins, which are poisonous to people with gluten intolerance

Often, doctors make no connection at all between patients' ailments and the consumption of wheat, even though a strict gluten-free diet alone can make many illnesses disappear and pounds melt away, as I have found in my coaching.

Wheat madness - my experiment: How white flour made me depressed

The link between white flour and mental illnesses

Observations from my coaching made me even more aware of white flour. Some of my coaching clients who had mental health issues loved white flour. They told me that they sometimes had episodes where they needed and ate pure white flour. Some would just mix it with sugar and eat it, others would mix the flour with water and sugar and drink the mixture or make pancakes. Especially for clients with severe mental disorders, such as borderline, flour products were almost like an addiction.

A client called me and said, "Dantse, I'm down again. I drank two cups of white flour mixed with water. I can't do it anymore. I'm scared. I want to kill myself." What role had the flour played in that? I don't know exactly. But with this woman, when she had an episode, somehow flour products were always "around."

Another client who suffered borderline personality disorder was able to tear an entire baguette loaf of white flour into pieces, dip it in plain oil, and eat it in just 15 minutes. White bread was as bad for her as the disease itself. These behaviors really got me thinking about researching the connection between wheat and mental illnesses like depression. I conducted an experiment on myself and also ate a lot of white flour, in all forms, including in pure form, like these clients. After 5 days, my mood totally changed. I actually had a depressed and aggressive mood. I felt generally unwell for no reason. I became more powerless steadily and found little drive to exercise, which I normally do enthusiastically.

I suddenly drank a lot of coke, drinks that I normally don't even drink once a year. But the thirst for carbonated drinks was very great, even for carbonated water. In those 5 days, my sugar and salt consumption also changed tremendously. What I really noticed very strongly was that I, a positive thinking person, was suddenly overflowing with negative thoughts and blaming third parties. I could hardly get out of my negative thoughts. This mood improved briefly when I started eating white flour again, but a short time later this nervousness and lack of drive intensified again.

I also felt a lack of desire for sex, because I started having problems with erection. I had migraines and headaches for hours for the first time in my life, as well as other complaints such as abdominal pain, difficult bowel movements, pimples, pain in the bones, sudden heart palpitations, and so on.

Remarkably, the symptoms magically began to disappear just one day later, when I stopped eating white flour and totally changed my diet. My erection also returned to normal. But I struggled a bit to escape the addiction to bread that was slowly setting in. I didn't notice, or rather observe, that I had gained weight until a few days later. It was clear to me after this experience, which I will detail in the book "Wheat Madness," that wheat - at least to me - was addictive, made me continue to eat poorly (more salt, sugar, butter, milk), made me physically ill, and perhaps psychologically? Unfortunately, there isn't much reporting on this, but the reports I found seemed to confirm my experiment and observations. White flour seems to be really addictive for certain people, just like cigarettes and alcohol. I have not yet been able to determine whether it is the disease that makes these people addicted to flour, or whether the white flour exacerbates or even causes their disease.

***

More and more scientific studies show that wheat is massively attacking our health, especially our thinking ability and memory. It insidiously destroys our brain and makes us dumber. The consequences can be chronic headaches, massive sleep disorders, dementia or Alzheimer's disease.

Dr. William Davis, cardiologist, shows in his book "Wheat Belly" (2011) how genetically modified wheat makes us addicted and can even control our thoughts and behavior. Through natural defenses, wheat prevents minerals from being optimally absorbed in the body. The result can be a change in metabolic processes, which can also be noticeable mentally.

Further processing with chemicals then makes it even more of a health hazard: wheat paunch, wheat addiction, obesity, spare tires, schizophrenia, abdominal pain, digestive problems, colon cancer, diabetes, heart attack, hyperacidity, fatigue, osteoporosis, high blood pressure and allergies are some diseases that can result from the consumption of wheat.

Like all foods that are rich in carbohydrates and starch, cereal products, such as bread or pasta, cause blood sugar levels to rise rapidly. As a result, the pancreas produces a lot of insulin, which causes premature aging of the cells.

Too much grain and grain products, or the mixture of grain and other industrial foods, not only make us sick, but also make us age faster.

People who eat little grain have a much nicer complexion. They have fewer wrinkles on their faces, their skin doesn't sag as quickly and their muscles aren't flabby.

Carcinogens in cereals (flour, rice, soy, corn, wheat, etc.), bread, refined flour

Cereals can also contain carcinogenic toxins, such as the herbicide glyphosate. In agriculture, however, this most commonly sold herbicide in the world is readily used to improve grain yield.

However, the plant toxin is suspected of damaging the genetic material in humans and animals and causing diseases such as cancer.

According to investigations by BUND and ÖKO-TEST, the herbicide was detected in the urine of 182 metropolitans from 18 European countries. Seventy percent of all samples in Germany are contaminated, i.e. the herbicide was present in the urine of seven out of ten metropolitans in Germany who were examined, according to BUND. This is proof that this active agent - contrary to the promises of the producers - is spreading through the food chain and that the population in Europe is largely contaminated with glyphosate.

In 2012, ÖKO-TEST had flour, oatmeal and baked goods tested for glyphosate and found it in 14 of 20 samples. Most notably, eight of the ten rolls tested were contaminated, proving that glyphosate survives baking temperatures.

A4.3 Refined and artificial sugars and cancer

Sugar can act like a poison. But the poison tastes so good and we make ourselves happy with our chocolate, our sweets, cake, ready meals, medicines, drinks, with our yogurt, ice cream, snacks and so on. Every day this poison ends up in adults and children, even in babies, although it is one of the biggest killers of all, as studies from the USA show. Up to 35 million people die each year indirectly from sugar consumption. Since wheat products become really delicious when sugar is added, sugar leads to excessive consumption of wheat. Sugar attacks baby teeth in children. Sugar is one of the main causes of obesity.

A high-sugar diet increases the synthesis of insulin (hormone storage) and decreases the production of glucagon (the hormone needed for breakdown), the antagonist of insulin. High insulin levels lead to weight gain. This weight gain lowers testosterone levels (confidence hormone and muscle synthesis). A low testosterone level also promotes weight gain!

Many sweets can adhere the vessels and be responsible for them aging faster.

Too much consumption of sugary food (sugar, sweets, cake, drinks, etc.) also attacks the skin. In a study published in the *British Journal of Dermatology,* researchers explain that sugar spreads proteins in the body that damage collagen and skin elasticity and accelerate aging.

Cancer loves sugar and especially industrial sugar (refined sugar). Industrial sugar is hidden in almost all convenience foods, soft drinks, baked goods, and baby and toddler foods, often under other names such as sucrose, syrup, fructose, glucose, lactose, maltose, or even just an E-number or chemical formula. Many products are advertised with the slogan "no added sugar" but contain fructose as an ingredient. This is a clear lie, as fructose is a sugar extracted from fruits. U.S. researcher Robert Lustig, who with his team conducted a study on the "toxic truth" of sugar (published in *Nature* Vol. 482 2012), said, "There is growing scientific evidence that fructose can cause quite a few chronic diseases and is toxic to the liver. [...] A little sugar may not be a problem, but a lot of sugar kills - albeit slowly."

Sugar makes you fat and cancer loves it where there is fat.

It has been scientifically proven that tumor cells need a lot of sugar to proliferate. Many researchers, such as Professor Lewis Cantley of Harvard Medical School suspect that in some cases, high sugar consumption causes cancer to develop in the first place. Sugar is a major fuel for cancer because the sugar causes a fermentation process to start in cancer cells that destroys surrounding healthy tissue and cripples the body's immune system, says cancer researcher Dr. Coy. And refined sugar (industrially produced sugar) drives insulin levels up even faster and also makes cancer cells grow much faster than with normal sugar.

Thanks to fructose, cancer cells can reproduce at lightning speed and spread throughout the human body, as scientists at the University of California, Los Angeles have proven in a study. Cheap syrup in drinks and ready meals consists of up to 90 percent fructose (corn syrup is preferred because it saves the industry a lot of money).

Sweeteners can be carcinogenic.

Aspartame was on the CIA's list of biochemical warfare agents until the mid-1970s.

Many sweeteners, such as aspartame E 951, cyclamate E 952 (banned in the U.S. since 1969), saccharin E 954, neotame E 961 and corn syrup (HFCS) are carcinogens. They are very popular in the industry because they are much cheaper than cane sugar and are contained in thousands of products - from soft drinks to chewing gum and baked goods to medicines.

Since aspartame rightly came into disrepute (carcinogenic), the industry developed neotame. But neotame is merely a much better, or rather a much worse aspartame. In the European Union, neotame was approved on Jan. 12, 2010, as a sweetener and flavor enhancer with the E number 961 for food. Since it is cheaper than aspartame, it is increasingly used by the industry. It is synthesized from aspartame and 3,3-dimethylbutyraldehyde and is 7,000-

13,000 times sweeter than sugar and 30-60 times sweeter than aspartame (E951). Some studies show that neotame is much more toxic than aspartame.

***** Sugar and simple carbohydrates are very carcinogenic*****

If you eat a lot of sugar, you should eat few carbohydrates (monosaccharides and disaccharides): "Because the fermentation metabolism in cancer cells depends on the supply of large amounts of glucose, a low-carbohydrate diet deprives the fermenting cancer cells of the basis for their aggressive, destructive behavior." And thus stop the malignant "TKTL1" cancer gene, according to Dr. Coy. But the Western diet in particular often consists of such mixtures of sugar and carbohydrates: Pasta, bread, cake, etc.

Almost all white flour products contain sugar and so we promote the development of cancer, its spread and because of fermentation the spread of metastases throughout the whole body.

A4.4 Meat: Overconsumption of animal protein may cause cancer

Excessive consumption of red meat and meat products such as sausage or cured meat can cause colorectal cancer, stomach cancer, and other forms of cancer such as lung and liver cancer.

Meat is not fundamentally unhealthy; the problem is much more the quality of the meat. In Africa, there are peoples who eat a lot of beef, like the northern Cameroonians. But they are fit, slim, muscular and live very long. Many nutrition experts warn against meat in general, instead of properly explaining why the meat is dangerous. It has only become more dangerous. Because good meat, in normal quantity - about 100 to 200 g - is very healthy for the body. If you eat too much of it, the meat can harm your health. However, the quality of meat has deteriorated because of the type of feed the animals got worse in quality. Animals that normally eat grass are fed grain that has been chemically and genetically treated and is full of pesticides.

Most processed meat products such as breakfast meats, bacon, sausages or hot dogs contain chemical preservatives that give them a fresh, appetizing appearance. The animals the meat comes from have been fed chemicals and genetically modified grains, which can cause cancer. In addition, nitrosamines can develop from the nitrite present in sausages.

Excessive consumption of meat can promote chronic inflammation, which can lead to conditions such as diabetes and other chronic diseases.

A4.5 Ready meals and frozen food

Ready meals and frozen foods are important sources of carcinogens in the body.

Some of this food is made almost entirely from artificial products. For example, some manufacturers use food imitations (pizza with cheese without milk, salami without meat). Ready meals contain too many dangerous preservatives, colorings, flavors and aromas, bad and too much fat and artificially produced sugar and are therefore a real cancer cocktail for the body. All the toxins I have covered so far and many more that we don't even recognize and can't track are in convenience foods.

The very dangerous plasticizer DEHP was also found in ready meal products and canned foods as well as in fat-containing seasoning sauces. According to a study, mayonnaise or jarred vegetables and fish are also more heavily contaminated.

Frequent consumption of deep-fried frozen foods may increase the risk of prostate cancer. Studies show that people who eat a steady diet of ready meals and frozen foods are more likely to develop cancer. A study from the U.S. showed that men who eat deep-fried frozen foods such as French fries, chicken nuggets or pastries baked in fat, such as donuts, at least once a week are 35 percent more at risk of prostate cancer than others who turn to these products at most once a month.

Those who eat more fast food and ready meals, desserts, hamburgers, McDonalds, cake, butter and chocolate croissants, cookies, etc., age faster and contract many diseases, including mental ones like depression!

Industrially processed food contains less useful and helpful nutrients for the body such as vitamins, minerals, zinc or folic acid, but instead too much sugar, too much bad milk, too much bad fat (trans fatty acids), too much acid, too much grain (wheat), too many chemicals (additives, hormones, preservatives, etc.) - all this destroys organs and cells and causes terrible diseases.

Fast food makes you age faster and can even lead to an earlier death. Especially because of the high phosphate content.

Phosphates are used as acidifiers in both food and beverages. The industry also uses them as acidity regulators, emulsifiers, as a melting salt, and as preservatives hidden behind the numbers E 338 and E 339. Too many phosphates cause various diseases such as arteriosclerosis and accelerate the aging process of the body and the early formation of wrinkles.

A4.6 Carcinogens in French fries, potato chips, popcorn, donuts

In French fries and chips, scientists from the Technical University of Munich have detected a substance that is "much more dangerous" than acrylamide - the highly carcinogenic glycidamide! Even the smallest amounts could cause mutations.

Acrylamide is formed during frying and was first detected in high quantities in food in 2002, according to the Federal Institute for Risk Assessment. In animal tests, acrylamide was carcinogenic.

The trans fatty acids in French fries can also be carcinogenic. Similar to donuts, French fries are deep-fried. Most fast food chains use hydrogenated fat. Trans fats thus end up in the fries or even in chicken wings. The risk of cancer increases. Trans fatty acids are formed during the industrial hardening of oils, such as in the production of margarines, baking or spreadable fats, but also during intense heating, such as deep-frying. Chemically hardened oils are popular with industry: they can be heated particularly intensely, they last longer and they are cheaper. Many countries have already banned trans fats or reduced their consumption. Trans fats not only increase the risk of cancer, they are responsible for many other diseases. They can even harm unborn children.

If the body takes in trans fats, they settle where unsaturated fatty acids (in nuts, fish) were intended. The trans fats replace the unsaturated fat purely physically, but they cannot fulfill the functions of the unsaturated fatty acids (such as cell function of the brain, the glandular function, oxygen transport). This leads to misunderstanding and impairment in the body, which ultimately causes harm.

The consumption of trans fats has a negative effect on the feeling of hunger. People who eat a lot of things that contain trans fats have the feeling that they are not quite full. This is because the body is not getting the fatty acids it needs. This leads to eating more, which in turn leads to weight gain. And obesity is one of the conditions that promotes cancer. Belly fat, in particular, promotes the development of cancer.

Chips, crackers, cookies, hard bread and fried onions should also be enjoyed with caution. In addition to sugar, these also contain trans fats, as in French fries and donuts. Unfortunately, trans fats are not listed on packaging, which would greatly protect consumers. Trans fats only have to be listed if the food contains more than 0.5 grams per serving, according to naturalnews.com. To avoid listing, manufacturers reduce the amounts listed until the trans fatty acid value is less than 0.5 grams.

Furthermore, white refined flour is used in the production of chips and cookies. This flour, like large amounts of sugar, is also harmful and promotes cancer.

Donuts

I have already written about a clear link between cancer risk and trans fats in French fries. Trans fats are used in the production of donuts. When hydrogenated fat is heated, artificial trans fats are created. Thus, there are vegetable oils that are hydrogenated to have a longer shelf life, their consumption increases the risk of cancer.

Popcorn

Microwave popcorn is convenient but can be dangerous: As Canadian chemists have now discovered, phosphate esters (PAPs), often found in fast food packaging and microwave popcorn, enter the human body where they are degraded to perfluorinated carboxylic acids (PDCAs). These substances are traceable in humans worldwide and are strongly suspected of being a possible elicitor for cancer.

A4.7 Bad oil, bad animal fat, trans fats

Fatty foods, saturated fats (trans fats), high-calorie foods, ready meals, fast food, frozen foods, bad oil, mayonnaise and salad dressings, animal fat, sausage, smoked foods, cured foods, offal, schnitzel, meatloaf, pizza, breaded foods, canned fish, etc. are dangerous to health.

Not all fat is the same. One helps and the other destroys: white fat gets the kilos up, brown fat gets them down. It even consumes energy. Fats consist of glycerol and fatty acids. They are very important as energy stores and donors, as cushions, for the stability of cells, for the formation of new membranes. They transport certain vitamins - A, D, E and K - through the organism. In addition, cholesterol is an important precursor for steroids. These steroids include sex hormones.

There are two types of fatty acids: saturated and unsaturated.

Saturated fats and trans fatty acids are called "bad" fats. They increase cholesterol levels and promote cardiovascular problems.

Saturated fatty acids are found in numerous convenience foods such as butter, cheese, cream and other dairy products, fatty meats, sausages, etc. They become solid at room temperature.

Unlike unsaturated fatty acids, the body can also produce the components of saturated fatty acids itself.

Trans fatty acids, also called trans fats, are according to Wikipedia "unsaturated fatty acids with at least one trans-configured double bond between two carbon atoms. In the human diet, they are found especially in industrially produced food, where they are formed by rearrangement of the cis double bonds into the trans configuration as by-products of the incomplete hardening of vegetable oil. Consumption of glycerol esters of trans fatty acids increases the level of LDL cholesterol in the blood. They are considered contributors to coronary heart disease (atherosclerosis, myocardial infarction)."

Trans fats increase the level of bad cholesterol and lower the level of good cholesterol.

Trans fats cause other diseases such as obesity, type 2 diabetes or Alzheimer's disease.

Trans fats often appear on the list of food ingredients as "hydrogenated vegetable oil". Hydrogenated vegetable oils - or trans fats - are oils that have been industrially processed. Hydrogen is added to the oil to harden it. Unlike natural fats, it does not go rancid even without refrigeration. As a result, foods appear less greasy.

Trans fats are found everywhere: in French fries, potato chips and all fried foods such as chicken wings, in cookies, Berliners and puff pastry, in ready-made soups, gravy, sausage, cereal bars or breakfast cereals.

A4.8 Fruit is good and healthy, but too much fruit can also make you sick and fat

Fruit is and remains the best and healthiest alternative when you're hungry in between meals - unlike a bar of chocolate or a piece of cake. But you should pay a little attention to the quantity.

Apple, orange, pear, mango, pineapple and co. are super healthy and delicious, but their consumption can unfortunately also have unpleasant consequences if you eat them too often. They can even make you fat, because carbohydrates and fructose are also hidden in the fruit. Moreover, fruit alone does not make you really full.

In addition, fructose (when present in large quantities) can cause a feeling of hunger in the brain or it does not cause the brain to tell us that we are full. Therefore, one tends to eat even more, even though one is not hungry. Thus, with fruit you can accumulate a lot of calories, acting against the good intention of losing weight.

Another danger are the chemicals with which the fruit is treated nowadays. Many of these chemicals interfere with fat metabolism. As I have mentioned many times before, the mantra "the dose makes the poison" also applies here.

A4.9 Diet food, light products and dietary supplements

Almost all scientific studies warn against diet foods, diet drinks and light products. Diet drinks, like Diet Coke, are worse for your health than regular sugar-sweetened soda. "Diet" soda and other diet drinks and foods may be carcinogenic.

All of these drinks, which are healthier at first glance, contain aspartame. Aspartame is a synthetically produced sweetener. As a food additive, it is declared as E 951. The substance is suspected of being highly carcinogenic. Aspartame is a widely used ingredient in many products such as soft drinks, confectionery, baked goods and dairy products.

From one aspartame diet soda per day, the risk of cancer increases!

The results of a recent aspartame study (a total of 77,218 women and 47,810 men took part in the studies, which ran over a period of 22 years) show: just one can of diet soda (coke light, iced tea without sugar, *sugarfree*, diet fruit spritzer or other light drinks) of 355 ml a day

- increases the risk of leukemia (blood cancer) by 42%.
- increases the risk of developing multiple myeloma (bone marrow cancer) by 102% in men
- increases the risk of non-Hodgkin lymphoma (cancer of the lymph glands) in men by 31

In each case, compared with control subjects who did not drink diet sodas.

Already in the past, independent scientists found that the consumption of aspartame can lead to various diseases such as cancerous tumors, lymphoma, leukemia, nerve damage, kidney failure, seizures and premature death.

Other substances, such as sucralose, supposedly derived from sugar, cause brain and nervous system dysfunction, migraines, cancer, and weaken the immune system.

The consumption of saccharin is also not recommended.

Many diet foods contain additives that help build fat in the body. It has been proven that fat promotes cancer. Even though aspartame, saccharin and the like don't provide calories, they still cause you to get fat. Since the body naturally holds on to its calorie account, it demands a second and a third after *one* light yogurt. And inevitably, you get fat.

The funny thing is that many products call themselves "diet" because they contain sweeteners instead of normal sugar and are therefore low in calories, but in no way lead to weight loss.

The NRW Consumer Center in Germany has found carcinogenic substances such as sibutramine or the probably carcinogenic phenolphthalein in many diet products and, although they were declared as purely herbal.

A4.10 Fat deficiency: too little good oil and too few vegetable fats

The prevailing oil phobia is a mistake and it is unfounded. In Africa, the fat from plants (i.e. oil) is used to cleanse the skin and keep it elastic.

Most people in Europe think that eating low-oil food would be healthier. However, the opposite is true. Our hormonal system needs fat to function well. People who consume little oil are therefore much more easily affected by hormone deficiencies. Our hormones, including sex hormones, need cholesterol. A deficiency in sex hormones leads to weight gain, irritability, loss of libido, chronic fatigue. The skin becomes drier and wrinkled, muscles become flabby and disappear. One looks older.

Oil deficiency can also cause mental illnesses such as depression.

American physician Andrew Stoll, a psychiatry professor at Harvard Medical School in the U.S. state of Massachusetts, blames the widespread lack of omega-3 fats for the spread of psychiatric illnesses. Depression, schizophrenia, even behavioral disorders are in part related to a lack of adequate good fats. In my coaching, I found that most people who came to me for psychological distress (they felt listless, lazy, powerless, always tired) used little or much less oil in their cooking than other, healthier people.

Oil deficiency can also promote cancer

In Cameroon, women were told to "Eat oil so you can have healthy breasts!"

My teacher told me that lots of good oil from plants would be a very effective prevention against breast cancer. Insufficient oil supply in the body would harm the fatty tissue in the breast area and cause the breast to be insufficiently supplied with oxygen, because fat not only serves as an energy provider in the body, but also helps oxygen to reach the cells.

When I studied some scientific studies, especially the research of Dr. Dr. Otto Warburg, Nobel Prize winner in 1931, I began to understand what my master had tried to explain to me. Because lack of oxygen in the cells can lead to development of cancer. The lack of oxygen in breast tissue could be very significant when it comes to cancer. But I could not find more detailed information and studies about it, with provable facts.

I strongly suspect that people who consume very little oil promote inflammatory processes in the body, because without oxygen, there is inflammation. And inflammation stimulates cancer cells.

A4.11 Acidic foods make you fat and sick: hyperacidity of the body is the cause of many chronic diseases and cancer

A diet excessively consisting of acidic foods is not good if you want to stay healthy. These foods are harmful to the body and therefore should be avoided or not consumed too often. Acid forming foods should always be mixed with alkaline foods so that they do not harm us.

"The body creates as many fat cells as it can during hyperacidity. Fat is ideal for storing acids or their waste products and at the same time protects the vital organs from the dangerous acids. You are possibly not fat at all, but simply overacidified! And as long as you are overacidified, a permanent weight loss often remains an unfulfilled wish. In an overacidified state, a diet is therefore not only useless, but also not very intelligent. You would be depriving your organs of their bodyguard and exposing them to corrosive acids." (Excerpt http://www.zentrum-der-gesundheit.de)

Hyperacidity makes you fat.

By the way, with an alkaline diet, the kilos often fall quite automatically.

You should quit

- dairy products such as cream, butter, cheese, cottage cheese. This will significantly strengthen your immune system. You will notice that certain ailments, such as migraines, headaches, flatulence and gastrointestinal problems, impure skin will disappear or will not be felt so intensely. We are talking about excessive consumption of dairy products. A little bit of it certainly does not disturb health. Humans are the only creatures that still drink milk in adulthood. This is not natural.
- ready meals and processed food: contains too many chemicals that make fat burning virtually impossible
- fast Food
- all low fat products and light foods
- high sugar food
- bland food
- cold food
- fat-free food (vegetable fat)
- cereal
- bad drinks and carbonated drinks

An overacidified body cannot lose weight and gives rise to many diseases, such as cancer, a healer from Cameroon told me. If the pH-value of the body is not in balance, you can't be fit. Cancer is also caused by too many acids.

This warning from my teaching in Africa almost 40 years ago is also confirmed today in modern science.

A4.12 Acidic food list

However, acid-forming foods do not taste acidic in every case. Only their effect on the organism is acidic. They make your body acidic. In turn, sour-tasting foods, such as some fruits, can belong to the alkaline foods.

Bad acid-forming foods include:

- Meat from conventional agriculture, chemicals
- Meat broth, sausages, ham
- Eggs from conventional farming
- Fish and seafood from conventional aquaculture or originating from polluted regions
- Milk and dairy products (curd, yogurt, kefir and all kinds of cheese, also from sheep and goat; especially all low-fat dairy products)
- Heavily processed soy products (especially textured soy protein, abbreviated TVP, which is offered in dried form as a base for ground meat substitutes, goulash substitutes, and the like).
- Cereal products made from superfine flours (bakery and pasta products such as cake, pastries, sweet pastries, noodles, etc., some breakfast cereals such as cornflakes, ready-to-eat cereal, crispies, crunchies, etc.)
- Products made from gluten (seitan), e.g. vegetarian sausages, cold cuts, bolognese or similar
- All products that contain sugar
- Sweeteners such as thick juices, but also honey

- Ice cream, including water, soy and yogurt ice cream - exception: alkaline ice cream
- Convenience products of all kinds, especially those from conventional production
- Ready-to-drink beverages such as soft drinks (e.g., lemonade, coke, etc.), fruit juice from concentrate, isotonic drinks, protein drinks, milkshakes, drinks for weight loss, etc.
- Mineral water and in generally carbonated drinks
- Tea (black tea, fruit tea, iced tea, etc., only herbal teas are alkaline, even highly alkaline).
- Products containing alcohol and alcohol
- Coffee, including cereal, instant and decaffeinated coffee and caffeinated products
- Mustard
- Vinegar
- Ketchup
- Acid preserves

With support from: http://www.zentrum-der-gesundheit.de.

*Honey can be integrated into the diet IF it comes from high quality sources.

A4.13 Water and mineral water

One cause of disease can be unclean water, but even clean, pure water can make you sick.

Do we know any animal that drinks carbonated water?

Anyone expecting a study from the industry that clearly proves that too much water, and especially water with carbonic acids, is unhealthy and can also make you fat, will quickly be disappointed if you take note of who the major mineral water manufacturers are: Nestlé, Pepsico, Coca-Cola and Danone.

Yes, mineral water can make you fat.

Many will be surprised, perhaps laugh at me or even shake their heads when I tell them that our favorite liquid, water, can make you fat.

In Africa they say that too much water makes you fat and sick, and indeed the first weight loss is water. Very early on in Cameroon, I learned that you have to trust your body's sensibilities. That means you drink when you are thirsty. A healthy body gets healthy impulses. I told my father at that time that we learned in school that you should drink at least 3 liters of water a day. My father, who passed on to me many wisdoms and secrets of nature, mind, body and spirit, showed me with simpler examples that there is no certain amount of water that can be prescribed to a person. Bodies and needs are too different, and it is important not to disregard one's body feeling with one's mind. You should drink when you are thirsty and not the other way around. You should not be forced or be badly reprogrammed. There is a clear connection between water and the tastes of sweet and salty. People who eat very sweet and very salty drink much more than people who eat spicy. The excess water that the body can no longer excrete, is stored in cells and this makes us fat. Another disadvantage is the increased excretion of minerals and vitamins, because of the more frequent need to urinate.

Water also makes you fat and sick because of plastic packaging. Most plastic packaging contains the chemical bisphenol A, a plasticizer that leaks from the plastic into the water and thus into our bodies. The water in plastic bottles has a very high estrogen concentration. This chemical affects fat metabolism and leads to obesity and diseases such as cancer and makes men infertile. Carbonated water in particular contains larger amounts of plasticizer because the carbonic acid aggressively attacks the plastic.

Carbonated mineral water seems to be very unhealthy for the body. We were always warned about this in Africa. I was always told that beer - also because of the carbonic acid in it - not only makes you fat, but also sick. I didn't even know that there was carbonated water. In Africa, or rather in Cameroon, there is only still water. Carbonic acid stretches your stomach, my nature teacher in Cameroon told me, so you eat a lot more. It gives you a false feeling of satiety that quickly disappears, making you eat more often.

Also, the plasticizers and chemical additives in drinks like coke, fanta, sodas, etc. make your body fat.

It is also believed that there are hormonal pollutants from birth control pills in tap water: Women excrete the hormones taken via the pill in their urine; these then enter the groundwater and cannot be filtered out. Thus, they get into the tap water and harm men in particular. In addition, bisphenol A, a dangerous hormone-like chemical, can be found in drinking water, which is released into the tap water via the coated drinking water pipes.

A4.14 Tea

Studies show that herbal teas can cause cancer. Pyrrolizidine alkaloids are present in high amounts in tea, herbal tea and dried medicinal plants. For children, pregnant women and nursing mothers, the harmful substances in herbal tea could be dangerous. Scientists are finding "unexpectedly high levels of pyrrolizidine alkaloids," or PAs, in herbal and other teas.

The Federal Institute for Risk Assessment warned in summer 2013 that many herbal teas are contaminated with carcinogenic substances! Children, pregnant women and nursing mothers in particular should not drink too much herbal tea. Adults who drink more than five cups of tea a day could do themselves a lot of harm.

In a study, the experts examined a total of 221 different commercially available herbal tea and tea samples as well as tea drugs (dried medicinal plants). These included baby fennel tea, chamomile tea, nettle tea, lemon balm tea and peppermint tea. High levels of the secondary plant compounds pyrrolizidine alkaloids (PA) were found in many of them, explained Andreas Hensel, president of the German Federal Office for Risk Assessment (BfR). Secondary plant compounds are substances that certain plants produce naturally as a defense against predators and microbial attacks and also act as growth regulators. Studies have shown that these substances cause cancer in animal experiments.

In an updated ÖKO-TEST (a few months later), 15 teas were examined. Two conventionally produced and even three organic teas contained pyrrolizidine alkaloids. Pregnant women, nursing mothers and children should therefore not only drink tea or alternate it with other beverages.

There are no legal limits for PA in food in Germany. Surprisingly, however, there is a legal limit value in the pharmaceutical sector.

A4.15 Coffee

Even though many studies and the food industry tell us that coffee is healthy, we should be careful, because it is not entirely true. In comparison, coffee can actually do more harm than good. Unfortunately, this rarely comes across. The caffeine in coffee is not always good for you.

Caffeine is actually an insecticide that the coffee plant produces to protect itself from insect feeding. The poison acts like a stimulant in humans. Coffee fights fatigue and keeps you awake. Have we asked ourselves why? It has to do with the stress hormone adrenaline. Caffeine increases the production of this hormone. It constantly puts our body in a state of emergency, as if a sudden danger or event appeared and we had to defend ourselves or flee, or as if we were in a competition. The consequences are: Increase in blood pressure, heart rate and muscle tone. But since nothing happens and we often just sit there, the situation soon turns. The kick passes and we fall into an extreme tiredness, exhaustion, nervousness, a general feeling of discomfort. Headaches can - occur.

Caffeine feigns stress, increases the noradrenaline level and reduces the serotonin level, a neurotransmitter with a calming effect. That's why you become more restless and fidgety. Coffee contributes to the development of depression or depressive feelings.

There is even a term for chronic poisoning by caffeine already: caffeinism, the addiction to coffee and the psychological and physical consequences of it. People who suffer from it often have anxiety and mood swings, are quickly irritable, dissatisfied, fall more often into depression, have eating disorders and suffer from insomnia, hyperactivity, concentration problems.

Is a single cup of coffee more carcinogenic than a pesticide?

Some experts even believe that coffee is more dangerous than pesticides. This opinion is expressed by the well-known U.S. biochemist Bruce Ames in "Dietary Pesticides (99.99% all natural: carcinogens/mutagens/clastogens/coffee)". He opines that caffeic acid has been shown to be carcinogenic when fed in large quantities to rats and mice. One cup of coffee contains 10 milligrams of caffeic acid. He compares this amount to pesticide residue levels of some carcinogenic pesticides in food, which is less than 10 milligrams over the whole year. Bruce Ames was a researcher at the Children's Hospital of Oakland Research Institute (CHORI) and was director of the National Institute of Environmental Health Science at the University of California, Berkeley.

A4.16 Pure juices

Pure juices and freshly squeezed juices are healthy, but can also make you sick. For orange juice, for example, many oranges are pressed, including the peel, and only then filtered. The problem is that the fruit itself has been sprayed and treated with various chemicals, such as pesticides, for weeks and months. Although they are washed, residues of these chemicals get into the juice and thus into our bodies, with the consequences we can imagine.

Juices can also pose a risk of diabetes if you drink a lot of them, according to several studies, as a 2013 Harvard School of Public Health study proved. The reason is the structure of fruit juices.

In the transition from fruit to juice, the fiber is lost and the fructose in the juice goes into the blood faster and completely, raising blood sugar more than if you eat the fruit.

In addition, many people have an intolerance to fructose (fruit sugar). More and more people suffer from it without doctors identifying the disease. For those affected, the ingestion of fructose is painful. The fructose ends up undigested in the large intestine and causes abdominal pain, flatulence, diarrhea, nausea and even depression, headaches, susceptibility to infections and a deficiency of certain micronutrients, such as folic acid and zinc, if the intolerance is not treated for years.

In case of fructose intolerance, the following foods are forbidden:

- Most fruits (grapes, oranges, apples, mangos, etc.) and all products from them.
- Dried fruit
- Honey, jam, chocolate, candy, etc.
- Convenience products that may contain sugar
- Diabetic products
- Sweeteners: they additionally inhibit the absorption of fructose from the intestine and consequently aggravate fructose intolerance

A4.17 Alcohol - highest cancer-promoting potential

Many diseases are caused or aggravated by the consumption of alcohol. There is an alcohol disease called "drunkenness", "alcohol addiction" or "alcoholism".

But you don't even have to be an alcoholic before alcohol makes your body sick. Excessive alcohol consumption damages the body in many ways. Long-term alcohol abuse leads to numerous chronic secondary diseases in addition to alcohol addiction and alcohol poisoning.

Alcohol harms

- the metabolic process and this can have these consequences:
    - Damage to the liver, leading to fatty liver, alcoholic hepatitis and cirrhosis, pancreatitis,
    - Cardiomyopathy, coronary heart disease and anemia
    - Sugar metabolism disorders, lipid metabolism disorder
    - Osteoporosis
- the mucous membranes in the mouth, throat, esophagus and stomach
- the brain and nervous system

Alcohol favors:

- Cancer of the nasopharynx and cancer of the larynx
- High blood pressure

- Mental disorders such as depression, delusions, anxiety
- Dementia and Alzheimer's disease
- Eye-muscle paralysis
- Inflammation of the optic nerves
- Inflammation of the pancreas
- Eating disorders and obesity
- Acidification of the body, cause of further diseases
- Impotence and listlessness
- Diarrhea
- Hormonal disorders

Further diseases include:

- Wernicke-Korsakoff's syndrome, it occurs when the body lacks vitamin B1. It can lead to movement disorders with paralysis, changes in character, delusions, dementia and nervous disorders
- Pure Korsakoff's syndrome is a form of amnesia (memory impairment)
- Hepatic encephalopathy is a potentially reversible brain dysfunction that results from inadequate detoxification function of the liver
- Alcohol poisoning

Babies are affected by maternal alcohol abuse while still in the womb and they show the typical facial features of fetal alcohol syndrome, are often intellectually disabled and their growth is delayed.

In addition, doctors in Cameroon strongly advise diabetics not to drink red wine.

A4.18 Carbonated sweet drinks such as coke and lemonades

In 2010, 184,000 people died from overly sweet drinks, including about 133,000 from diabetes, 45,000 from heart disease and 6450 from cancer.

The consumption of sugary soft drinks, such as coke and soda, isotonic drinks, energy drinks or protein drinks not only makes you fat, it also causes many diseases such as diabetes, cancer, metabolic syndrome, cardiovascular problems, etc.

Coke contains about 42 calories (kcal) per 100 milliliters, and a 0.5-liter bottle contains the equivalent of 18 sugar cubes.

According to many studies, these sugary and chemical containing drinks accelerate the aging of the body's cells almost as much as smoking.

Two glasses of lemonade a day harm the body just like smoking!

One of the main reasons is the high phosphate content. In soft drinks and sweet pop drinks as well as lemonades, phosphates are mostly used as acidifiers, acidity regulators, emulsifiers, melting salts and preservatives (E338, E339).

Depending on the consumption, the body can even age by years because of that. A study by the University of California published in the *American Journal of Public Health* has proven this. Prof.

Elissa Epel and her colleagues established a possible link between sugar drink consumption and cellular aging. Many results showed that consumers of carbonated sweet drinks had shorter telomeres.

Researchers found that people who consume at least 350 milliliters of sugary soda drinks a day are physically 4.6 years older than people who stick to water or tea. In addition, the risk of developing pancreatic cancer increases from two glasses per week. Energy drinks often contain three times the amount of caffeine as coke. The carbonic acid also releases more plasticizers from the plastic bottles and thus enters the blood - with all the consequences I describe in the following chapter. We have already read a lot about sweet drinks, such as coke and co. We know that they are unhealthy, but we don't really know what exactly happens to our bodies.

What happens in your body in the first 60 minutes after drinking a can of coke?

During my research, I came across the following information, which for the first time exactly explains in detail what coke does to our bodies. The British health blogger Niraj Naik has listed on his website "The Renegade Pharmacist" what a can of cola does to the body within just one hour. This example shows how fructose and carbonated drinks destroy us more and make us fatter than the so-called saturated oils.

The original text (own translation) comes from: http://www.blisstree.com/2010/06/23/mental-health-well-being/what-happens-to-your-body-if-you-drink-a-coke-right-now/

"According to Niraj Naik, when you drink a can of coke or a similar sugary and caffeinated beverage, here's what happens in your body....

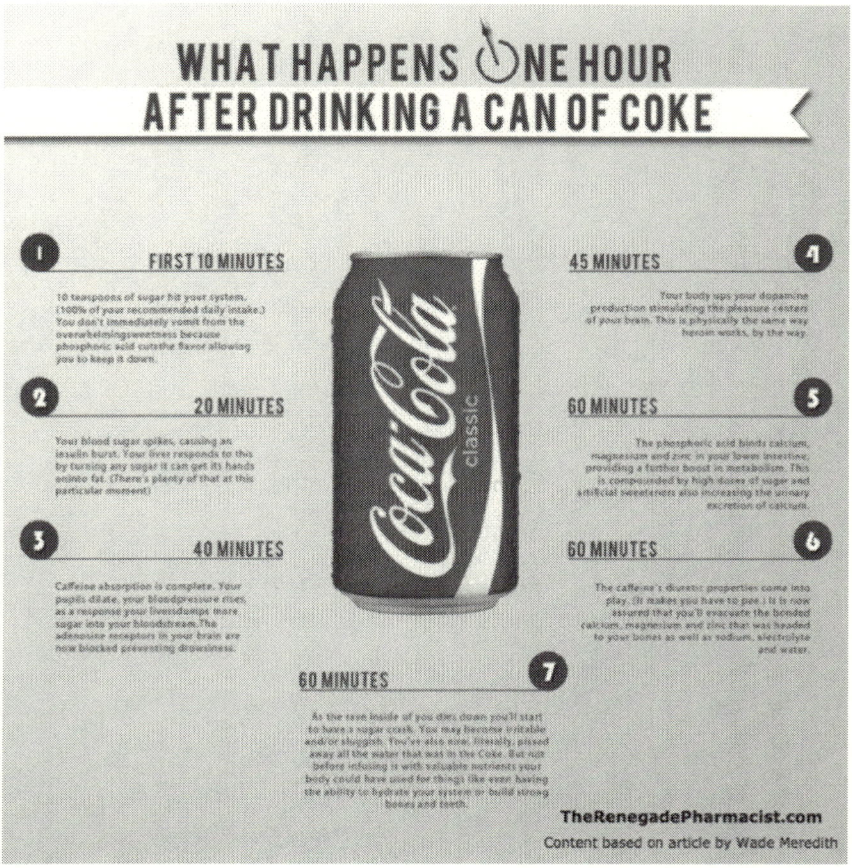

http://therenegadepharmacist.com/wp-content/uploads/2015/05/coke1hr3.jpg

1. **In the first 10 minutes**: Your body is flooded with 10 teaspoons of sugar (that's 100% of the recommended daily intake.) The only reason this overwhelming sweetness doesn't make you nauseous is because phosphoric acid mellows the taste.
2. **20 minutes**: Your blood sugar peaks, causing the release of large amounts of insulin. Your liver responds by converting any sugar it gets its hands on (and there's more than enough of it right now) into fat.
3. **40 minutes**: You've now completely absorbed the caffeine and it's having its effect: your pupils constrict, your blood pressure rises, and in response, the liver dumps even more sugar into your bloodstream. The adenosine receptors in your brain are blocked, which prevents drowsiness.
4. **45 minutes**: Your body increases dopamine production, which stimulates the brain's reward center - the same way heroin works, by the way.
5. **60 minutes**: The phosphoric acid binds calcium, magnesium and zinc in the intestine, thereby boosting metabolism. This is further driven by the high sugar content and artificial sweeteners - meaning even more nutrients end up in the urine.
6. **60 minutes**: The diuretic properties of caffeine kick in: You have to go to the bathroom and excrete the calcium, magnesium and zinc that your bones should have. Your body also loses sodium, electrolytes and water.
7. **60 minutes**: The roller coaster ride in your body slowly comes to an end and the sugar level in your blood plummets: you become tired and irritable. And you have now flushed all the water contained in the coke down the toilet, after your body has enriched it with all the valuable nutrients.

In the next few hours (if you are a smoker probably after 2 hours at the latest) the caffeine crash will follow.

It is not specifically coke that is the enemy, but the explosive mixture of extremely high levels of sugar, phosphoric acid and caffeine - and this is found in almost every soft drink. We should actually all know the health risks of these drinks, because the mixture of sugar, carbonated water and additives such as phosphoric acid and salt produces far too much acid in our bodies.

A glass now and then doesn't do much damage; as always, the right amount is critical."

A4.19 Synthetic salt

Without salt we can do nothing, it would hardly be possible to move the body and even think, because it contains very important minerals and trace elements. But you can live well without salt, if you can absorb these minerals elsewhere, for example from herbs, fruits, nuts, meat, wild plants and so on.

But not all salt is the same. Natural salts are rarely found in Western foods. Most of the salts we buy in the supermarket are industrially processed. They are refined, which means they are bleached, boiled and purified. The industrial salt, mostly pure sodium chloride, still has hardly any important minerals such as potassium, magnesium, selenium, etc., these have been replaced by chemicals, such as aluminum (hydr)oxide, potassium hexacyanidoferrate(II)), fluorine compounds, iodine, etc.

Artificial iodine in food makes you sick.

Iodized foods are found almost everywhere in the Western diet: bread, many dairy products, because animals are fed iodized mineral feed mixtures, sausages, convenience foods, fast food, chips, some sweets, pastries, eggs, because chickens are fed iodized feed, and even soil vegetables, because soil is contaminated via the excretory products from animal feed.

Many people get sick from iodine without knowing what is causing it. Occurring diseases can be: Asthma, impotence, acne, -conjunctivitis, heart disorders, sleep disorders, depression.

Salt and ntrosamines: Too much salt promotes cancer development

Where does the iodine actually come from? The iodine that is added to salt comes from saltpeter mixtures and recycled materials such as printing inks, catalysts, X-ray contrast agents and disinfectants.

Table salt causes cells to die, causes diseases such as kidney stones, bladder stones, gallstones, gout, arthrosis, arthritis to develop and promotes cellulite. It is suspected that Alzheimer's disease, thyroid disease, high blood pressure, brain and heart disorders are also promoted by industrial salt.

The fluoride in salt is also a health hazard. Certain forms of bone cancer are said to be favored by excessive fluoride intake, according to http://www.zentrum-der-gesundheit.de.

Table salt also contains nitrites (sodium nitrite), which can form nitrosamines with proteins. Nitrosamines are among the most aggressive carcinogens. Many sausage and meat products contain sodium nitrite. And now you understand why people warn against eating a lot of meat.

Healthy salts are for example: Fleur de Sel, the most precious and expensive sea salt, rock salt and crystal salt.

A5 Low vitamin diet is the cause of many ailments and cancer: a list of ailments depending on vitamin deficiency.

Name	Deficiency
Vitamin A (retinol)	Growth arrest, night blindness
Provitamin A **Beta carotene**	Accelerated aging process
Folic acid	Increased risk of cancer, fatigue, digestive problems, nervousness, poor memory, insomnia, confusion, miscarriages, shortness of breath
Vitamin B1 (thiamine)	Severe muscle and nerve disorders, fatigue, digestive disorders, dropsy, heart failure, cramps, paralysis, tingling in arms and legs
Vitamin B2 (riboflavin)	Skin inflammation (rare), brittle fingernails, anemia, corneal opacity
Vitamin B3 (**niacin**, nicotinic acid)	Skin and mucous membrane inflammation, headache, tremor, sleep disorders, dizziness, depression, tingling and numbness

A5 Low vitamin diet is the cause of many ailments and cancer: a list of ailments depending on vitamin deficiency.

Name	**Deficiency**
	in the limbs.
Vitamin B5 (**pantothenic acid**)	Nerve dysfunction, poor wound healing, early graying, weakened immune system
Vitamin B6 (pyridoxine)	Intestinal problems (rather rare), bad skin, fatigue, brittle corners of the mouth
Vitamin B7 (**biotin**, vitamin H)	Fatigue, skin inflammation, muscle pain, hair loss, nausea, depression
Vitamin B9 (**folic acid**, vitamin M)	Anemia, digestive disorders, hair, bone and cartilage growth disorders
Vitamin B12 (cobalamin)	Anemia, nerve disorders, nervous disorders, changes in the lungs and spinal cord.
Vitamin C (ascorbic acid)	Bleeding gums, fatigue, joint pain, headache, poor wound healing, lack of appetite, scurvy, poor performance

A5 Low vitamin diet is the cause of many ailments and cancer: a list of ailments depending on vitamin deficiency.

Name	Deficiency
Vitamin D (calciferol)	Bone curvature and softening, osteomalacia, increased susceptibility to infections, muscle weakness
Vitamin E (tocopherols)	Visual impairment (rare), fatigue, muscle wasting, unpleasure, reproductive difficulties
Vitamin K (phylloquinones)	High doses of vitamins A and E counteract vitamin K

(*** With the help of Jumk.de)

A6 Low mineral diet causes many diseases: List of ailments, depending on mineral deficiency

The human body cannot be healthy without minerals. Doctors attribute the cause of many diseases to a lack of minerals.

Name	**Deficiency**
Boron **B**	Bone diseases, growth problems, arthritis, fungal and bacterial infections
Calcium **Ca**	Bone decalcification, poor dentition and bone structure, allergies, high blood pressure, migraines, heart problems
Chloride **Cl**	Premature hair and tooth loss
Chromium **Cr**	Irritability, depressiveness, -hypoglycemia, high cholesterol, anxiety, diabetes
Iron **Fe**	Anemia, poor hearing, menstrual pain, restless legs syndrome, fatigue
Iodine **I**	Thyroid problems, goiter, tough mucosa

Name	Deficiency
Potassium **K**	Vomiting, drowsiness, muscle weakness and paralysis, low blood pressure, drowsiness, confusion, extreme fatigue
Copper **Cu**	Anemia, edema, bleeding, problems with skin pigmentation, hair problems, easy irritability, loss of sense of taste, loss of appetite
Magnesium **Mg**	Irregular pulse, lack of drive, kidney stones, asthma, osteoporosis, depression and anxiety, PMS, period pain, fibromyalgia, glaucoma, diabetes, low endurance (especially in athletes), insomnia, migraines, gum problems, high cholesterol, high blood pressure, hearing loss, prostate problems
Manganese **Mn**	Dermatitis, poor memory function, epilepsy, anemia, diabetes, heart trouble, arthritis
Molybdenum **Mo**	Male impotence, easy irritability, irregular pulse

A6 Low mineral diet causes many diseases: List of ailments, depending on mineral deficiency

Name	Deficiency
Sodium **Na**	Sunstroke, drowsiness due to heat
Phosphorus **P**	Confusion, lack of appetite, weakness, easy irritability, speech problems, decreased resistance to infections, anemia
Selen **Se**	Decreased immunity and resistance to infections, decreased fertility in males, age spots, retarded growth
Vanadium **V**	Not known
Zinc **Zn**	Male infertility, skin rash, arthritis, ulcers, growth problems, allergies, alcoholism

*** Thanking www.orthoknowledge.eu/vitamine-tabel/

A7 Plastic packaging: Plastic parts in food

Much plastic packaging is highly contaminated with toxins. The most common endocrine disrupting chemicals found in plastic include phthalates and bisphenol A (BPA).

The chemical compound **BPA**, the starting material for polycarbonate and epoxy resins, which is also added to plastics such as polyamide, silicone or latex, is said to have significant effects on men's fertility. The substance acts in a similar way to the female sex hormone estrogen. BPA, which is used to harden plastic, is one of the most widely used industrial substances with global sales in the billions. The substance is found, among other things, in food packaging, food cans (are lined on the inside with a thin plastic layer. This is almost always made of epoxy resins, which release BPA into the food), in dental fillings, CD cases, building materials or in the lining of some baby bottles. In almost all chapters of this book, I have to talk about plasticizers - that's how common and dangerous they are.

Phthalates are found as plasticizers in various plastics, mainly PVC, polycarbonate (PC), etc.

Phthalates and bisphenol A are traceable in human blood, urine, breast milk and umbilical cord blood of newborns and they are very potent carcinogens.

We also find plasticizers in many sweets, Nutella, butter, cheese or whipped cream. An estimated 40 percent of our food contains toxic plasticizers. This was the conclusion reached by the NDR household program "The big kitchen check”.

There was a big shock in 2010 when the German Federal Environment Agency identified the dangerous plasticizer DEHP, a phthalate, in Nutella. DEHP is one of the most dangerous plasticizers of all. Even then, the Federal Environment Agency had tested 600 children for the plasticizer. The result: every child was contaminated with DEHP. The values of some children were classified as extremely alarming by toxicologists who were consulted. In addition to suspected carcinogenic effects, studies have shown that plasticizers can attack the sex organs of men and make them infertile.

A8 Chemicals and poison in organic farming

Generally, it is said that organic products (meat, vegetables, fruit and co) mustn't be genetically modified and mustn't contain chemical fertilizers or pesticides. Unfortunately, this is not always the case.

Organic is not always organic. Not all organic products are the same. Especially the organic brands of the supermarkets can contain carcinogenic substances. Dioxin has already been found in organic eggs!

Many organic products are sprayed with pesticides just like conventional products.

One danger with organic products is mold. To combat this, conventional poisons are sprayed, which unfortunately can be found in some organic products at the end-consumer.

Dangerous additives are also used in many organic products; it is therefore very important to read the ingredient list on the packaging carefully. Some have been proven to be carcinogenic, and the consumer needs to know that organic products may also contain up to seven additives without labeling. This means there can be the same additives in organic products as in conventional products, but they can still be called "organic."

- Carrageenan: found in organic dairy products. Carrageenan is extracted from red algae and is extremely controversial, as the substance has led to ulcers and changes in the immune system in animal tests
- Nitrite curing salt: certain organic sausage products contain nitrite curing salt, which can form carcinogenic nitrosamines

- Ascorbic acid (vitamin C)
- And many more

In Germany, organic associations such as "Demeter" do not use such dangerous additives.

In the past, carcinogenic substances have repeatedly been found in organic products. The consumer organization Foodwatch warned about acrylamide in some organic potato chips: Acrylamide is carcinogenic.

Another case occurred in 2007, when Stiftung Warentest (leading German consumer safety group) found a particularly high concentration of the carcinogenic substance benzopyrene in "Bio Negro" dark chocolate. Benzopyrene belongs to the carcinogenic group of substances known as polycyclic aromatic hydrocarbons (PAHs). The product was withdrawn from the market at that time.

In 2013, Stiftung Warentest found the potentially carcinogenic substance anthraquinone in Pura Pesto from Basilico Genovese D.O.P. with a best-before date of July 4, 2014.

A9. Free radicals

Heart disease, cancer and rheumatism have something in common: free radicals. These are broken parts of molecules with a so-called unpaired electron in the atom of the breaking point. The free radicals are aggressive in their search for their missing electron and in the process, they destroy other substances, cell membranes, chromosomes or tissues.

Free radicals are formed during all metabolic processes in the body, such as stress or immune defense, inflammations, injuries, high physical stress, but also by external influences such as tobacco, UV radiation, X-rays or food additives such as preservatives, colorants, flavorings as well as herbicides, fungicides, pesticides and nitrates. Certain drugs, smog, exhaust fumes, air pollution, dioxins, methane, ozone, solvents, heavy metals, body care products also promote the formation of free radicals.

Free radicals cause inflammations in the body. These inflammations are important because it is a normal and helpful reaction to neutralize these aggressive radicals. Therefore, small amounts of free radicals are not a problem for the body. In larger amounts, when the body cannot adequately break down the free radicals, oxidative stress occurs. The body's ability to defend itself is overloaded, which leads to the death of cells and membranes and the development of chronic diseases.

Many studies have confirmed a link between an abundance of free radicals and the aging process, as well as the occurrence of degenerative diseases such as heart disease and stroke, cancer and atherosclerosis, dementia and Parkinson's disease.

A9. Free radicals

Aging is partly explained by the wear marks caused by the reactive atoms and molecules - the free radicals.

We would be able to live healthier and young longer if we reduced the level of free radicals or neutralized them.

A10 Inflammations are also caused by an unhealthy diet

Inflammations occur to protect the body from invaders such as bacteria, pollutants and so on. Inflammation is therefore a natural defense mechanism of the body.

In many chronic diseases such as cancer, Alzheimer's disease, osteoporosis, bronchitis, diabetes, etc., inflammatory reactions occur in the body. Inflammation can be recognized by various signs: Fever, redness, spots, pain, swelling, etc.

Besides viruses, fungi, environmental toxins, bacteria, stress and lack of exercise, the cause of **inflammations** can also be poor nutrition: Over-acidifying diet, refined sugar, white flour, dairy products, ready meals and microwave food, additives in food, bad drinks such as coke, fanta, soda, etc. and a diet low in vital substances such as vitamins and minerals.

When the acid-base level in our body is disturbed, our body will show inflammatory reactions more often. The intake of additives changes the intestinal flora, which promotes inflammations.

With an anti-inflammatory diet consisting of alkaline foods rich in vitamins and minerals (vitamins A, C and E, trace elements such as selenium, zinc, magnesium, etc.) and omega fatty acids, we can protect our body from many inflammation-related diseases.

A11 Tables of morbid, carcinogenic and hazardous additives in foods

In today's modern diet, disease-causing additives have become a normality that many people are not even aware of, but which causes most diseases in our bodies. If these additives and chemicals were reduced, many people would not even go to the doctor. Artificial flavors, colors, glutamate and preservatives negatively affect our health and make us sick. Additives are responsible for many chronic inflammations in the body.

20 percent of Germans suffer from lactose intolerance. This also has to do with these chemicals, because some additives can trigger allergies and food intolerances, such as lactose or gluten intolerance.

Preservatives from chemical structures can be recognized by the E-numbers 200-299 to. All food additives are labeled with E numbers. The "E" stands for "Europe".

There are currently more than 300 different additives.

This table only includes food additives that are considered to be of concern or dangerous. In addition, some substances used in foods and food supplements that have not been approved as food additives and therefore do not have an E-number are listed at the beginning.

It is recommended, especially for risk groups such as allergy sufferers and young children, to make an individual assessment of which substances would like to or should be avoided.

As always, the phrase "the dose makes the poison" applies, but since we eat or drink several foods at the same time, this dose is reached quite quickly.

A11.1 Table of hazardous dyes (E 100-180)

Food colorants are food additives that are used to make food look better and to satisfy consumers' color expectations. They also serve to compensate for color losses due to processing and can therefore feign better quality under certain circumstances.

Bold = substances that are particularly hazardous and/or harmful even in small doses

E-No.	Name	Hazard
E 100	Curcumin	Dysfunction of the thyroid gland, allergenic
E 102	**Tartrazine**	**Allergenic, suspected of causing ADHD in children**
E 104	**Quinoline Yellow WS**	**Allergenic, suspected of causing ADHD in children, further effects largely unknown, banned in the USA (suspected of causing cancer)**
E 110	**Sunset Yellow FCF, Orange Yellow S**	**Allergenic, probably asthma- and neurodermatitis-inducing, suspected of causing ADHD in children, caused kidney tumors in animal tests**

A11 Tables of morbid, carcinogenic and hazardous additives in foods

E-No.	Name	Hazard
E 120	Cochineal, carminic acid, true carmine	Allergenic (rarely)
E 122	**Azorubine**	**Side effects on blood count, lungs, lymphatic system, pancreas, suspected of causing ADHD in children**
E 123	**Amaranth**	**Carcinogenic, allergenic (probably also asthma and neurodermatitis), in animal experiments caused calcium deposits in the kidneys, banned in the USA, not to be confused with the quinoa**
E 124A	**Ponceau 4 R, Cochineal Red A**	**Allergenic, suspected of causing ADHD in children**
E 127	**Erythrosine**	**Impairs nerve and especially thyroid function, is discussed as a cause of hyperactivity in children, carcinogenic, promotes ulcer formation**
(E 128)	**Red 2 G**	**Carcinogenic, allergenic, approval currently revoked**
E 129	**Allura Red AC**	**Scarcely studied, allergenic, suspected of causing ADHD in children**
E 132	Indigotine, indigo	May affect digestive enzymes,

E-No.	Name	Hazard
	carmine	rarely allergenic
E 142	**Green S, Brilliant acid green BS**	**Suspected of causing Alzheimer's disease, mutagenic in animal studies**
E 151	Brilliant black BN, Black PN	Allergenic
E 154	**Brown FK**	**Damage to liver and heart, staining of almost all organs colored by unknown metabolites of E154, allergenic**
E 155	**Brown HT**	**According to the EU Scientific Committee on Food, contains "about 20% of an unidentified added dye", is stored in kidneys and lymphatic system**
E 160A	Carotenes, beta-carotene	Increased risk of lung cancer in smokers and people with cardiovascular disease when intake is high
E 161g	**Canthaxanthin**	**Damage to eyes and liver, assessed as a "risky substance" by the German Federal Health Agency**
E 171	Titanium dioxide	No significant research to date in terms of impact
E 173	Aluminum	Suspected of causing Alzheimer's disease, accumulated in the body

E-No.	Name	Hazard
		by kidney patients
E 174	Silver	Blocks a variety of enzymes, deposits in tissues
E 175	Gold	May cause blood picture disorders
E 180	**Lithol Rubine BK**	**In animal tests: increased mortality, causes hyperactivity, various side effects on kidneys, spleen, thyroid and infection defense, allergenic**

A11.2 Table of hazardous preservatives in food (E 200-298)

Extend the shelf life of food.

E-No.	Name	Hazard
E 210	**Benzoic acid**	**High toxicity, causes allergies, asthma, hives, can cause epileptic seizures in high doses, forms carcinogenic benzene in the presence of ascorbic acid (E300)**
E 211	**Sodium benzoate**	**see E210**
E 212	**Potassium benzoate**	**see E210**
E 213	**Calcium benzoate**	**see E210**

E 214-219	**PHB ester**	**Allergenic, inducing convulsions in animal tests**
E 220	Sulfur dioxide	May cause headaches, asthma attacks, allergies and nausea, breaks down vitamin B1
E 221-228	Sulfites	see E220
E 230	**Biphenyl, Diphenyl**	**Promotes bladder cancer, internal bleeding and organ changes in animal tests, caused deaths in manufacturer's works,** approved for peel treatment -> gets onto flesh when peeling with fingers (citrus, bananas)
E 231, 232	**Orthophenylphenols**	**see E230**
E 233	**Thiabendazole**	**Damage to liver, kidneys, spleen, heart, cancerous changes in the thyroid gland, now only listed as a pesticide, but use remains the same: peels of citrus fruits and bananas, see also E230**
E 234	Nisin	Concerns about the formation of resistant pathogens

E 235	Natamycin	Antibiotic drug, pathogen resistance to be feared due to use in foodstuffs
E 239	**Hexamethylene tetramine**	**Breaks down highly toxic, highly carcinogenic formaldehyde, reacts with protein to form unexplored modified protein**
E 242	Dimethyl dicarbonate	Decomposes immediately into carbon dioxide and methanol as well as possibly into toxic methyl carbamate, reacts with food ingredients, no labeling requirement (!)
E 249-252	Nitrates and Nitrites	Can react in stomach and intestine or when heated above 130° (meat roasting/grilling) to form carcinogenic nitrosamines, toxic, acutely dangerous for small children because oxygen transport is blocked
E 270	Lactic acid	D-lactic acid cannot be broken down by infants. Acidification of the blood may occur. However, only L(+) lactic acid is permitted for infant foods.

E 280	Propionic acid	Cancerous changes in the forestomach in animal experiments, banned in Germany in 1988, now permitted again in Germany by the EU
E 281-283	Propionate	see E280
E 284, 285	**Boric acid & borax**	**Accumulate in the body as toxins, organ damage, used to cause poisoning, therefore now only approved for caviar, no antidote known**

A11.3 Table of dangerous antioxidants in food (E 300-321)

These ensure that food stays fresh and edible for longer and retains its flavor and color. Antioxidants make food last longer but can also serve as a stabilizer or emulsifier.

E-No.	Name	Hazard
E 301	Sodium L-ascorbate	Promotes bladder cancer, in animal experiments: growth impairment of young animals, often declared simply as "ascorbic acid" like E 300
E 310	Propyl gallate	Can lead to cyanosis in infants, impaired the

E-No.	Name	Hazard
		defense against infections in animal experiments, possibly allergenic
E 311	Octyl gallate	see E310
E 312	Dodecyl gallate	see E310
E 315	Isoascorbic acid	Suspected of preventing the absorption of natural vitamin C (ascorbic acid)
E 316	Sodium isoascorbate	see E301, hardly any studies
E 319	Tert-buthylhydroquinone	Allergenic, suspected carcinogenic effect
E 320	Butylated hydroxyanisole (BHA)	May be carcinogenic, accumulates in fatty tissue, enters the fetus, decomposition into substances when heated, whose health safety has not been confirmed, changes in immune system, blood count, liver and thyroid, allergenic
E 321	Butylated hydroxytoluene (BHT)	see E320

A11.4 Table of dangerous emulsifiers, stabilizers, thickeners and gelling agents in foodstuffs (E 322-495)

Emulsifiers combine two immiscible liquids, such as fat and water, to form a stable emulsion. Stabilizers are used to keep texture, flavor, or other properties stable. Thickeners are substances that are primarily capable of binding water. Gelling agents swell in water and gel.

E-No.	Name	Hazard
E 325-327	Lactate	see E270
E 338	Orthophosphoric acid	Suspected of causing osteoporosis, calcification and hyperactivity, contains significant arsenic, cadmium and uranium residues, often declared as "phosphate", impedes absorption of calcium, magnesium and iron
E 339-343	Phosphates	see E 338
E 385	**Calcium disodium ethylene diamine tetraacetate (EDTA)**	**May greatly increase the absorption of heavy metals**
E 400	Alginic acid, alginate	May interfere with the absorption of various minerals (calcium, magnesium, manganese, iron, zinc)
E 401-405	Alginates	see E 400

E-No.	**Name**	**Hazard**
E 407	Carrageenan	Changes in the immune system and ulcers in animal tests, allergenic, tumor hazard not conclusively clarified
E 407A	Processed eucheuma seaweed	see E 407
E 412	**Guar gum**	**Often heavily contaminated with hazardous substances, damage to esophagus, stomach and intestines, impairs digestion, alters intestinal flora, promotes flatulence**
E 413	**Tragacanth**	**WHO assumes that Tragacanth is "a massive allergen, capable of causing extremely severe reactions"**
E 420	Sorbitol, sorbitol syrup	Can lead to cramps relatively quickly
E 425	Konjac, konjac gum	Impedes the absorption of various nutrients

E-No.	Name	Hazard
E 432-436	**Polysorbates**	**Reactions during production not foreseeable, suspected of making otherwise non-absorbable substances absorbable**
E 442	Ammonium phos-phatides	Assessment for health unresolved
E 444	Sucrose acetate isobutyrate	Health assessment unresolved, in dogs liver and bile damage, is almost never declared
E 450-452	Di-, Tri- and Poly-phosphates	see E 338
E 476	**Polyglycerol polyricinoleate**	**Damage to liver and kidneys in animals, maximum dose can be exceeded very quickly**
E 491	Sorbitan monostesrate	Toxicologically not independently evaluated
E 492-495	Sorbitol-fatty acid compounds	see E491

A11.5 Table of anti-caking agents and acidity regulators in foodstuffs (E500-586)

Anti-caking agents are adherents to prevent lumping by the consumer. Acidity regulators keep the desired pH value of a foodstuff constant.

E-No.	Name	Hazard
E 503	Ammonium carbonate (hartshorn)	Harmful to health if eaten directly, ammonium disappears during baking, but E 503 is also approved for unbaked foods
E 510	**Ammonium chloride (salammoniac)**	**Alteration of parathyroid glands, adrenal cortex and blood count, bone damage, in pregnant women: hyperventilation, loss of appetite and vomiting**
E 512	Zinc 11 chloride	May cause nausea and vomiting
E 520-523	Aluminum sulfates	see E173
E 540-544	Other di-, tri- and polyphosphates	see E 338, for E 541 (sodium aluminum phosphate) see also E 173
E 554-559	Aluminium silicate	see E 173
E 586	4-Hexylresorcinol	Toxicologically controversial

A11.6 Table of dangerous flavor enhancers and glutamates in food (E 620-650)

Enhance the flavor of dishes, saving manufacturers expensive, high-quality ingredients.

E-No.	Name	Hazard
E 620	Glutamic acid	May cause "Chinese restaurant syndrome" in sensitive individuals (headaches, nausea, stiff neck), in animal studies: learning problems in the offspring and reproductive disorders, increases appetite and thus supports obesity
E 621-625	Glutamates	see E 620, partly also contained in yeast extract
E 626	Guanylic acid	Is converted to uric acid in the body, hardly any studies
E 627-629	Guanylates	see E 626
E 630-636	Inosinic acid and Inosinate	see E 626

A11.7 Table of hazardous sweeteners in food (E420, E 900-1520)

These are synthetically produced or natural substitutes for sugar that significantly exceed its sweetening power. They sweeten beverages and diet products in particular, but can be found in almost all convenience foods, fast food products, ice cream, etc.

E-No.	Name	Hazard
E 420	Sorbitol, sorbitol syrup	Can lead to cramps relatively quickly
E 950	Acesulfame-K	Carcinogenic in animal experiments
E 951	**Aspartame**	**May cause headaches, memory loss, visual disturbances, drowsiness and hyperactivity. Some studies classify this chemical as carcinogenic**
E 952	**Cyclamate (mostly sodium cyclamate)**	**Banned in the USA since 1969 because of suspected causing cancer. In animal experiments, damage to testicles and sperm by degradation products**
E 954	**Saccharin**	**The sodium salt used causes bladder cancer in animals, appetite stimulant, harmful in bladder diseases due to drug interactions**

E-No.	Name	Hazard
E 958	Glycyrrhizin (licorice)	May cause headaches and cardiac arrhythmias
E 959	Neohesperidine DC	Still unexplained, appetite stimulant
E 960	Neotame	Succession development of aspartame (E 951)
E 962	**Aspartame-acesulfame salt**	**see E 950 and E 951**

A11.8 Table of pollutants, toxins and carcinogenic substances in food: Where do they occur and what diseases do they cause?

Poison	Occurrence	Explanation
Acrylamide	Chips, French fries, speculoos	Mutagenic, liver-damaging, probably carcinogenic. Acrylamide is also converted in the liver to the far more dangerous glycidamide
Agaritine	Raw mushrooms, dried mushrooms	Carcinogenic
Alcohol (ethanol)	Beer, wine, high-proof alcohols	Carcinogenic. Liver-damaging in large quantities. Highly addictive.

A11 Tables of morbid, carcinogenic and hazardous additives in foods

Poison	Occurrence	Explanation
Anthraquinone	Partly contained in black tea. Partly in very questionable quantities.	Carcinogenic substance possibly formed during production process. Unresolved.
Antibiotics	Meat, seafood from aquaculture, dairy products	Promotes resistance to antibiotics and the emergence of super-resistant bacteria
Aluminum	Naturally present in many foods, or via canned foods and aluminum kitchen utensils. Elevated levels in pretzels, tea.	Damages the brain. Possibly responsible for Alzheimer's disease
Arsenic	Seaweed, fish, especially maties, seafood, especially mussels, rice, especially wholemeal and parboiled rice	May cause skin cancer, liver cancer with regular intake
Aspatarme	Sugar substitutes, sweets, diet products	May contain toxic impurities. Always contains toxic methanol. Suspected to be carcinogenic. E-number: E-951

Poison	Occurrence	Explanation
Azo dyes	Candy, brightly colored food	Very questionable, carcinogenic dyes. Partly they contain: Benzidine. E numbers: E 102, E 104 (quinoline yellow), E 123, E 129, E 180
BHT	Desserts, chewing gum	Interferes with blood clotting, suspected cancerous, may cause allergies. E number: E 321
Benzene	Partly in soft drinks, various food products	Benzene is carcinogenic. Can be formed if ascorbic acid or vitamin C is present in the beverage in addition to benzoic acid.
Benzoic acid / sodium benzoate	Preservative. Naturally present in berries, blueberries, mushrooms. Extends shelf life of food. Partly contained in soft drinks.	Carcinogenic, can cause ADHD, headaches, digestive problems, allergy. In combination with ascorbic acid: can produce carcinogenic benzene.
Bisphenol A (BPA)	Plastic food packaging, plastic kettles (!), partly thermal paper, plastic kitchen containers, house dust, food cans	Acts like hormone. Has a negative effect on fertility. May cause ADHD. Suspected cancer!
Cadmium	Dark chocolate, nuts,	Carcinogenic, nerve

A11 Tables of morbid, carcinogenic and hazardous additives in foods

Poison	Occurrence	Explanation
	spinach, celery	damaging, bone damaging. Originates from the natural composition of cultivated soils.
Cholesterol	In animal fats, especially in pork	Excessive intake promotes arteriosclerosis, increases risk of heart attack and stroke
Coumarin	Cinnamon cookies, woodruff	Harmful to liver, carcinogenic.
Cyclamate	Sugar substitute in diet products, sweets	Unresolved suspicion of causing cancer
Fungicides	Especially on citrus fruits & strawberries	Shall prevent fungal infestation of food.
Hardened fats	Margarine, convenience products, sweets, etc.	Accumulate in fatty tissue and are not broken down
Genetically modified food	Many vegetables and cereals affected. Must be declared in the EU if over 1% in food. No declaration requirement for animal feed for meat/dairy products.	Partly contain excessive pesticide load or unknown poisons. Impairs ecological agriculture, promotes patents on living beings!

Poison	Occurrence	Explanation
Saturated fatty acids	Especially in animal fats, coconut fat	Have an unfavorable effect on cholesterol levels. Increased risk of heart attack and stroke.
Glutamate / flavor enhancers	Ready meals, snacks, Chinese dishes, yeast extract. Also occurs naturally in vegetables.	May cause intolerance in some people. Mild neurotoxin. E number: E 621
Glycidamide	French fries, potato chips, highly heated foods.	Formed during the digestion of acrylamide. Highly carcinogenic and mutagenic. Amounts in food are small.
Glyphosate	Widely used active ingredient in many pesticides for "crop protection".	Most important chemical herbicide (weed control). One of the brand names is "Roundup".
Histamine	In red wine, alcoholic beverages, canned fish (especially tuna), in cheese (the older, the more), sausage/ham and sauerkraut.	Is a toxic substance, does not need to be declared. May cause headaches and "hangover". Harmful to blood and heart. Very problematic for histamine allergy sufferers.
Melamine	Plastic, which is often used to make tableware.	By heating melamine tableware (from 70°C), melamine and

Poison	Occurrence	Explanation
		formaldehyde get into the food. Risk of cancer and kidney disease.
Methanol	Main component of so-called fusel oils in alcohol. Partly also in fruit juices	Damages the nervous system. May cause blindness in higher doses. Toxic.
Mineral oil (MOSH / MOAH)	In various foods, e.g. edible oils, chocolate. Also through "staining" of cardboard recycling packaging and printing inks.	Mineral oil is harmful to health (including liver damage). However, due to contamination in the soil, during processing, through the packaging can not always be avoided.
Sodium nitrite, nitrite curing salt	In heated and then warm stored spinach, in highly heated cheese/sausage, and in cured foods.	E numbers: E 249; E 250; E 251; E 252. Preservative. Other names for comparable substances: potassium nitrite, nitrate, potassium nitrate. Inhibits oxygen uptake of the blood.
Sodium fluoride Fluorine	In table salt, in Anglo-Saxon countries partly also added to tap water.	Is very toxic. Supposedly of essential importance for dental health.

Poison	Occurrence	Explanation
Natamycin	Antibiotic-like substance in the rind of conventionally produced cheese. E 235.	May co-induce antibiotic resistance.
Nitrate	In drinking water, in various vegetables such as spinach, lettuce (in winter), chard and arugula (in winter).	Can be converted to carcinogenic nitrosamine in the stomach.
Patent blue	In food as a blue color.	Rather harmless. May cause allergies.
PET bottles: Acetaldehyde/ Estrogen	PET bottles are often used as packaging for beverages.	Acetaldehyde, which is harmful to the liver and cells, is released from the plastic into the beverage. In addition, estrogen-like hormones are often found in the contents of the bottles.
Phthalates	Plastic food packaging	Phthalates dissolve through fat or liquids and pass into food. They are found, for example, in soft films around sliced cheese or in coatings on food cans.

A11 Tables of morbid, carcinogenic and hazardous additives in foods

Poison	Occurrence	Explanation
Phytoestrogen	Soy / tofu products, beans	Hormone-like effect, cancer-promoting in some women at extremely high levels of consumption.
Polycyclic hydrocarbons (PAH)	Grilled and smoked foods	Formed during incomplete combustion and are carcinogenic. Partly contained in black teas.
Pyrrolizidine alkaloids	Occurs partly in herbal teas (especially chamomile, lemon balm) and honey and in arugula.	Is a natural component of plants toxic to humans. Extremely toxic substance!
Radioactivity	Occurrence in food: Wild meat, wild mushrooms, goods from contaminated areas (e.g. Fukushima, or Pacific). Also due to uranium partly contained in mineral waters.	Beware of wild mushrooms, seaweed, tuna.
Saccharin	Sugar substitutes, sweets, diet products	Unresolved suspicion of causing cancer in large quantities.
Safrole	Nutmeg, camphor,	Toxic

Poison	Occurrence	Explanation
	rootberry	
Mold toxin / Aflatoxins etc.	Cereals, bread, pistachios, peanuts, coffee, tomatoes tarnished brown (blight).	Harmful to liver, carcinogenic
Melting salts, phosphates	Processed cheese, cheeseburger etc. E 450 to E 495 (sodium phosphates, potassium phosphate, calcium phosphate etc.)	Damages kidneys, destabilizes bones, overall harmful effect. Life-threatening for kidney patients.
Semicarbazide	Plastic coated lids of beverages and food jars	Harmful to health. Acts like a hormone.
Silicones	Silicone additives in frying oil, especially in fast food chains. Name: E 900	The silicone itself is not toxic (although of concern because it is petroleum-based), but it multiplies acrylamide levels in fried products.
Solanine	Poison in the stem of the tomato, in immature tomatoes, in potato shoots.	Weak Poison.

A11 Tables of morbid, carcinogenic and hazardous additives in foods

Poison	Occurrence	Explanation
Stevia	Sweet drinks and sweets	Considered relatively harmless if not eaten too much. Maximum amount: 2g /day.
Sulfites	Wine, spirits, dried fruit, potato products	Health concern. Sodium disulfite destroys vitamin B1 in the body. Also problematic for allergy sufferers.
Trans fatty acids	Microwave popcorn, fried baked goods, puff pastry, French fries, potato chips, cookies (especially in products with "hydrogenated fats").	Harmful to health. See saturated fatty acids.
Vanillin	Confectionery, ready meals, in tobacco products	Artificial vanilla flavoring. Slightly harmful to health. Carcinogenic in large quantities or when burned.
Caramel coloring (ammonium sulfite)	Coke, drinks, sweets, whisky, jams	Sulfite ammonium caramel (E 150d) is contained in coke and is considered problematic. Inducing convulsions in animal experiments. Contains the carcinogenic

Poison	Occurrence	Explanation
		substance 4-methylimidazole.

With support from Christopher Stark, www.gesundheitstabelle.de

A12 Other pollutants: Nitrate, nitrite, dioxins, PCBs and metals

Nitrite, nitrate

As early as 1969 it became known that nitrite (for example E252 or E251) is present in foods, especially in meat, cheese and fish, which can lead to nitrosamines in the stomach. Many pharmaceuticals also form nitrosamine compounds with the nitrite from food, which are extremely effective carcinogens.

Dioxins and the dioxin-like polychlorinated biphenyls (PCBs). These chlorine-containing substances are very toxic and carcinogenic. More than 80% of the total intake occurs through food, such as meat, fish, eggs or milk, where the maximum limit is regularly exceeded. However, these cases are often not even known. Or only when it is too late and the contaminated products are already on the market and consumed.

Dioxins are colorless and odorless organic compounds containing carbon, hydrogen, oxygen and chlorine. According to Wikipedia, PCBs are toxic and carcinogenic organic chlorine compounds that were used until the 1980s primarily in transformers, electrical capacitors, in hydraulic systems as hydraulic fluids, and as plasticizers in paints, sealants, insulants and plastics. Dioxins such as PCBs are fat-loving and in some cases very persistent. They accumulate in the fatty tissue of humans and animals. Since dioxins and PCBs love fat, the risk of humans ingesting these substances increases with the fat content of the food. They hardly break down once they are stored in fatty tissue. With continuous ingestion of the toxins, the content in the body increases the older one gets, and so does the risk of cancer.

Metals

The most dangerous carcinogenic **heavy metals** that can be found in food are lead, cadmium and mercury.

Lead accumulates in bones and teeth and is particularly damaging to the nervous system and the hematopoietic system. In animal experiments, lead has also caused cancer.

Cadmium is preferentially stored in the kidneys, but also in other organs such as the liver or thyroid gland, as well as in the bones. Especially near busy roads and industrial plants, the concentration and intake of cadmium becomes very significant. Cadmium mainly causes lung cancer.

Mercury is mainly ingested through the consumption of fish and seafood, mostly in the form of organic mercury compounds. Mercury compounds have shown carcinogenic effects in animal studies.

Arsenic used to be used in paints and pesticides, for example. Today it is found in the workplace. Arsenic can cause lung cancer and, more rarely, skin cancer, and possibly other tumors, e.g. of the bladder.

Chromium, nickel and cobalt can also be found in food and can be carcinogenic.

A13 List of the most common diseases caused by poor nutrition

Two-thirds of all diseases in Western countries are linked to poor nutrition and an unhealthy lifestyle, scientists suggest.

Diet-related diseases occur in the following disease groups:

- Allergies
- Airways & Lungs
- Eye diseases
- Autoimmune diseases
- Musculoskeletal system, such as osteoporosis
- Blood diseases
- Hereditary diseases
- Erectile dysfunction
- Cold and flu
- STDs
- Skin diseases
- Heart disease
- ENT complaints
- Infectious diseases
- Cancer
- Circulatory diseases like high blood pressure & arteriosclerosis

A13 List of the most common diseases caused by poor nutrition

- Liver & gallbladder diseases
- Stomach & intestinal diseases
- Neurological conditions
- Mental suffering
- Rheumatic complaints
- Back problems
- Sleep disorders
- Metabolic diseases like diabetes
- Addiction
- Dental complaints

A14 Obesity: Diseases caused or aggravated by obesity

Being overweight is not just a visual problem. Obesity also endangers health. Too many kilos promote the emergence of many diseases and are the source of very many diseases such as:

- Diabetes mellitus type 2
- Gallbladder diseases
- Hypertension
- Eating disorders
- Lipopathy
- Back pain
- Osteoarthritis
- Respiratory diseases, such as sleep apnea
- Gout
- Breathing difficulties
- Heart diseases
- Cancer (uterine, breast, cervical, prostate, gallbladder)
- Sex hormone disorders
- Thrombosis and adiposity

Obesity also leads to psychological disorders such as depression, which in turn cause further illnesses. Not to be forgotten are psychosocial effects (exclusion, shame, lower recognition), which can lead to a reduction in self-esteem – which are all factors that promote disease.

B. Diet-related cancer

B1. What is cancer?

Cancer is the term used to describe pathological changes in cells. They cause cancer cells to divide more frequently and faster than healthy cells. They multiply uncontrollably, resulting in a bandage of degenerate cells. These malignant neoplasms grow into neighboring healthy tissue and destroy it. They migrate from their place of origin via the blood or the vascular system (lymphatic system) to other organs and multiply there as tumors, so-called metastases. (onmeda.de)

The older a person gets, the less reliable the repair system of the genes works. This is reflected in the number of new cases: the median age of onset for men and women is 69. However, there are also types of cancer that affect younger adults in particular. These include testicular cancer, for example: the median age of onset here is 38 years. (German Cancer Aid)

According to current knowledge from the U.S. National Cancer Institute, approximately one-third of all cases of cancer are attributable to diet.

Europe accounted for a quarter of all new cancer cases in 2012. The USA accounted for a fifth. The Middle East accounted for only about 8%, and Africa for a little less. The fact that diet also promotes the development of cancer was shown by the example of Japan and today, China. Almost 7 million of 14 million new cases were diagnosed in Asia in 2012, mainly in China and Japan. China is leading the way in Asia since they are adopting more and more of the Western dietary style.

B2 What can cause cancer?

One third of all cases of cancer are caused by the wrong diet: an unhealthy lifestyle with few fruits and vegetables but lots of animal fat (watch out: especially dairy products), drinks like soda pop and diet products, etc. The results of a recent study (http://lex.referata.com/wiki/Krebs) show the following: Even one can of diet soda of 355 ml a day - compared to control subjects who did not drink diet sodas - leads to

a. -a 42% higher risk of leukemia (blood cancer) in men and women,

b. -a 102% higher risk of multiple myeloma (bone marrow cancer) in men and

c. -a 31% higher risk of non-Hodgkin's lymphoma (cancer of the lymph glands) in men

Other factors that contribute to the development of cancer are:

- Chronic inflammations: Almost one in five cancer cases is caused by chronic inflammations. These inflammations are caused by hereditary factors, viruses, parasites, bacteria, pollutants, poor nutrition.
- Obesity, which in turn has to do with diet. Higher insulin levels increase the risk of cancer, as this hormone promotes cell growth.
- Being underweight can also stimulate the disease. A body with very little fat prevents nutrients from being absorbed well and that the transport of oxygen is ensured. Thus, the body cannot effectively fight free radicals and cell oxidation.

- Familial factors: In 5-10% of cases, the changes are hereditary. In affected families, cancer occurs in every generation and at a young age. According to current knowledge, cancer itself is not hereditary, but the predisposition to it can be inherited. This is known for breast cancer, colon cancer and ovarian cancer.
- Radiations: Intense UV radiation, ionizing radiation such as radon or X-rays, radiation accidents at nuclear power plants, etc., sun exposure.
- Chemicals, environmental toxins.
- Chronic infections, e.g. hepatitis B.
- Psychological factors? Scientists are very divided on this. Apparently, there is still no scientific evidence that personality traits directly trigger cancer or that depressed people are more likely to develop cancer than others. But psychological factors can still play a role in the development of cancer via unhealthy lifestyles.
- Poor lifestyle and living conditions: tobacco smoke, alcohol, lack of exercise and lack of physical activity.
- However, there are still numerous types of cancer whose elicitors are not known.

B3 Cancer in numbers: Rapid death rates because of cancer - Western countries are most affected

World Cancer Report 2014.

The number of cancer patients is rising rapidly worldwide

"Cancer is one of the greatest scourges of mankind, and a universal cure is not in sight. On the contrary: by 2015, the number of people who develop cancer each year will rise sharply," warns the WHO - and calls for stricter laws.

By 2025, 20 million people worldwide could develop cancer each year - around 40 percent more than at present. This is the conclusion of a study by the World Health Organization (WHO). In the next two decades, an increase of around 70 percent is possible. In 2012, there were around 14 million new cases of cancer, according to the World Cancer Report 2014, and around 8.2 million people died of cancer. In the next two decades, the number will rise to up to 13 million," according to focus.de from Monday, 03.02.2014, 14:03.

Germany:

In 1950, 493,416 people died in the Federal Republic, 80,841 of them as cancer victims; in 2011, the figure was 221,000. Almost three times as many.

The number of new cancer cases increased by 21% in men and 14% in women between 2000 and 2010.

In 2010, 477,300 people in Germany were newly diagnosed with cancer (252,400 men and 224,900 women), according to a recent estimate by the Center for Cancer Registry Data at the Robert Koch Institute. The most common forms of cancer among men are prostate cancer with 65,830 and lung cancer with 35,040 cases, while among women it is breast cancer with 70,340 and colorectal cancer with 28,630 cases (9th edition of "Cancer in Germany"). A total of 218,258 people died. Around one in four deaths in Germany is therefore attributable to cancer.

Scientists expected about 500,900 new cancer cases in 2014.

B4 Special environment that favors cancer development

Inflammations in the body is a welcome environment for free radicals. They trigger a cascade of reactions in the body, which in turn cause cancer-causing cell mutations. Susceptibility to cancer is a common cause of cancer, according to Professor Curtis C. Harris of the U.S. National Cancer Institute in Bethesda, "a pathological consequence of certain inflammations and the associated ongoing free radical stress and resulting DNA damage."

Inflammation is often due to a wrong and bad diet (industrial food, ready meals, milk and dairy products, refined sugar, trans fats, additives, genetically manipulated food, etc.). An acidic environment promotes inflammation and is poison if you want to fight cancer.

An unhealthy intestinal flora is an environment that promotes cancer development. More about this in Part A Chapter 3. "Intestinal disorders and an unhealthy intestinal flora".

Inflammations damage the cells and if these are not repaired in time or the damage is intensified by other influences (migraine, allergies, alcohol, cigarettes, etc.), cancer develops. More about this in part A chapter 9. about "free radicals".

Also, supplying the body with too little oil can have the effect of stimulating certain types of cancer, such as breast cancer. See Part A Chapter 4.10.1 "Oil deficiency can also promote cancer".

B5 Overweight and underweight promote cancer development

Cancer is significantly influenced by obesity. Overweight people are particularly susceptible to cancer. People who are overweight are more likely to develop the following cancers: uterine cancer, kidney cancer, gallbladder cancer, cervical cancer, thyroid cancer, blood cancer, liver cancer, ovarian cancer, breast cancer.

To this end, increased fat levels can lead to increased secretion of digestive juices. These juices contain bile acid, which can cause the intestinal flora to produce substances that lead to colon cancer.

Being underweight can also promote cancer. Severe underweight can lead to deficiency symptoms. The body is insufficiently supplied with vital nutrients: Fatty acids, amino acids, vitamins and minerals. Muscle and fat tissue are broken down, disrupting the active metabolism of the cells. The immune system is weakened. The fight against free radicals becomes difficult and the cells oxidize faster. Inflammations and infections are thus favored. Thus, many chronic diseases and cancer get the chance to develop well or to intensify and spread more. Therefore, it is also very important for cancer patients to be careful not to lose too much weight.

B6 Which foods promote cancer?

In my opinion, besides the well-known bad foods - like hot dogs, fries, chips and the like - **dairy products** are the foods that promote cancer the most. In a survey I did a year ago, when I was writing the book on cancer, I found that 80% of people who suffered from cancer had a huge consumption of dairy products and especially cheese. Coincidence? I honestly don't believe so, because all the people in my circle of acquaintances who suffered from cancer also ate a lot of cheese. I assume there is a correlation, but since dairy products are components of the industrial diet in almost 100% of cases, the studies will constantly contradict each other. We understand why.

Trans fatty acids: These are substances that are always formed when food is further processed in the factory and fats are hardened in the process.

Acrylamide: It is found in all foods that contain many carbohydrates and are heated to high temperatures, for example in French fries.

Here is a small list of foods that are carcinogens:

- Acidic foods
- Very many dairy products, whole milk and whole milk products such as cream, cream curd, crème fraîche, high-fat cheeses (> 30% fat content), yogurt, salted curd preparations, normal salted cheeses, processed cheese, butter, milk drinks, etc.

- Alcohol: beer, wine, liquor and much more. If you consume alcohol regularly, your blood pressure can increase in the long run. The alcohol causes blood pressure-increasing stress hormones and messenger substances to be released
- Fatty and high-calorie food, saturated fats (trans fats), ready meals and fast food, frozen food, bad oil, regular consumption of mayonnaise and salad dressing, animal fat, sausage, smoked foods, cured foods, offal, cutlets, meat loaf, pizza, breaded food, canned fish, etc.
- French fries, chips, donuts and other fried cereal products: They form substances such as acrylamide or glycidamide, which are carcinogenic
- Fish and seafood: Traces of arsenic can often be detected in them. Too high a dose of the toxin in the body can trigger skin cancer and liver cancer
- Raw mushrooms. They often contain agaritine, a substance that has been shown to be carcinogenic in animal tests
- Microwave popcorn
- Some varieties of black tea, because of questionable levels of pollutants.
- Cured meat products: they almost always contain sodium and nitrates, which are converted into nitrosamines when heated (for example, on pizza). Highly carcinogenic
- Hot dogs, because of nitrates. Nitrates are harmless, but in cooperation with the protein (amines) from the meat they form nitrosamines
- Foods rich in cholesterol

- Carbonated and soft drinks of all kinds, such as coke, lemonades, soft drinks, sweetened beverages, but also water (plasticizers). They contain the toxic substance benzene, which is formed when beverages contain ascorbic acid or vitamin C in addition to benzoic acid. Benzene is carcinogenic
- Excessive consumption of flour products
- Excessive consumption of sugar and sweets. They drive up insulin levels very quickly and promote the growth of cancer cells
- Ready meals with their numerous preservatives, colorants and other additives
- Hardened fat (trans fats), saturated fats. They change the structure and flexibility of cell membranes throughout the body
- Diet foods and drinks
- Unwashed fruit, such as grapes, apples, strawberries. They are contaminated with carcinogenic pesticides
- Fish oil increases cancer risk
- Not a food, but still related to food: eating too hot. I learned in Africa that "eating too hot" is not good for the body, because it can damage cells.

B7 Carcinogenic chemicals and toxins in food, households, agriculture

Many foods are carcinogenic. You can't see the harmful effect on the food and that's why they are such a problem. Of course, the majority of manufacturers try not to point this out to customers.

Tricks are used to deceive the consumer. Everything is done to hide some dangerous substances in our food. The legislator does not protect people as it should. For example, some dangerous toxins in food do not even have to be mentioned if they do not exceed certain limits, although they have been scientifically proven to have dire consequences for health. In order not to have to declare such substances, manufacturers reduce the quantities stated until they are below the limit. One example of this is trans fats in potato chips and cookies, although trans fatty acids are carcinogenic.

The great danger of food lies not only in the food itself, but in the added chemicals (additives, fertilizers, pesticides, etc.) and the way the agricultural products are processed. Many sources of cancer can be found in modern agriculture, animal breeding and factory farming, and the food processing industry.

In summary, humans poison themselves in several ways:

- Directly through the chemicals in agricultural products,
- By the chemicals and substances used to process these products into various food products,
- Through meat of the animals that were fed with the agricultural products

- Through meat of the animals bred with chemicals (such as hormones) and drugs
- Due to meat that has been processed with additives and other chemicals
- Through artificially produced food
- Through genetically modified food
- In addition, there is also poisoning by chemicals in the beverage industry
- Due to the interaction of individual substances in one or more products simultaneously

B7.1 Carcinogenic additives in food

Food additives: harmful or harmless?

According to official and regulatory information, the additives approved in the EU and Germany are harmless. Nevertheless, there have been heated discussions for ages about whether certain additives pose health risks. These discussions are fueled by studies that prove that some additives are dangerous, even if these studies are contradicted by others.

Many foods contain additives that are intended to improve the properties of food (color, sweeten or preserve). They can be identified on food packaging under "Ingredients", often abbreviated with the so-called E-numbers.

"According to current knowledge, approved additives are neither carcinogenic nor do they pose any other risk to health," says the German Cancer Center on its website, but it means those additives used within the prescribed limits in the EU.

But what about food produced elsewhere? Who controls the maximum limit? The authority or the manufacturer's declaration? Why have many of these substances been classified as carcinogenic and banned in other countries? What are the consequences if these different substances are found at the same time in a product or encounter other chemical substances? What chemical reactions happen and what new, perhaps toxic substances are then created?

An expert, who does not wish to be named, told me in a telephone conversation: "The interaction between the additives among themselves on the one hand and between the additives and other chemicals in the food on the other hand can lead to major health risks". It has been proven, for example, that the approved preservatives sodium benzoate and ascorbic acid or vitamin C can produce the carcinogen benzene, or that the preservatives E 252, potassium nitrate, and E 250, sodium nitrite, interact with protein building blocks to produce nitrosamines, a highly carcinogenic chemical.

The expert went on to say, "Maybe individual additives are not dangerous within limits, but then what if the maximum limit is exceeded? And no one can rule that out, and we even have to assume that there are such cases on the market." Here, too, it seems the phrase “quantity makes the poison” applies.

Azo dyes, colorants with the numbers E 102 to E 155 in the list below, are among the most harmful groups of colorants of all. Azo dyes approved for use in foodstuffs enter our bodies primarily through colorful confectionery and beverages. They are made from aniline. This has long been suspected of causing cancer.

List of food additives with E numbers that are classified as carcinogenic in some studies and countries but are permitted in Germany.

I have read many studies and researched in different countries. From these I have created a summary. Not all substances are listed, there are certainly more carcinogenic substances!

- **E 102 Tartrazine,** dye, hazardous, colors food lemon-yellow. Approved for: like E 110, banned in Austria, Finland, Norway, Switzerland.
- **E 104 Quinoline Yellow,** dye, hazardous, produces different shades of yellow. Together with blue coloring substances it is used to color food green. Approved for: same as E110. Suspected of causing cancer. Banned in the USA and Australia.
- **E 110, Sunset Yellow FCF**, colorant. Permitted for: Pastries, mustard, paracetamol, spirits, fruit wines (max. 200 mg/l), sherbet powder, sherbet, syrup (max. 50 mg/l), ice cream, jams, marmalades, fruit preparations, puddings, desserts. A carcinogenic effect was found in animal experiments. The substance is banned in the USA and many other countries.
- **E 120, Cochineal (Carmine)**, colorant also called carminic acid. Among food additives, the only colorant of animal origin. Very dangerous for children. Approved for: sweet drinks, chewing gum, yogurt, spirits, fruit wines, edible coatings for cheese and sausage, jams, marmalades, fruit preparations. The colorant carminic acid can be obtained from the louse by extraction. If carminic acid is mixed with aluminum salts, carmine is produced. According to the EU, carmine may only rarely be used today, and then mainly in

alcoholic beverages, as well as in cosmetics (lipstick), pharmaceuticals, and the textile industry.

- **E 123 Amaranth,** a dangerous azo dye, is banned in many countries such as the USA (since 1976) or France. Very hazardous chemical. Suspected carcinogenic effect. Amaranth may only be used in: Caviar (max. 30 mg/kg), liqueurs, wines and spirits (max. 30 mg/l). In addition, the dye is used in medicines, cosmetics and textiles.
- **E 124, Cochineal Red A**, dye, very hazardous chemical, colors food red. Approved for: same as E129, also ketchup, edible cheese rinds and sausage casings, sauces, condiments, chutneys (500 mg/kg), salmon substitute, surimi (500 mg/kg). The substance has been classified as carcinogenic by ARTAC, an association of doctors and therapists against cancer in France. The substance is banned in many countries such as the USA, Norway and Finland.
- **E 127 Erythrosine** is a dye and colors food pink to red. Permitted for: Cocktail cherries and candied cherries (max. 200 mg/kg), sweet cherries (Bigarreau cherries) in canned fruit (max. 150 mg/kg). It is also used as a colorant for pharmaceuticals and cosmetics. In the form of an aluminum lacquer, the red dye is widely used in lipsticks, for example. Suspected of promoting thyroid cancer.
- **E 128 Red 2G,** colorant for sausage and minced meat. In animal testing, this substance has caused genetic mutations and cancer.
- **E 129 Allura Red AC**, dye, belongs to the group of azo dyes. Approved for: Meat, pastries, confectionery, ice cream, puddings, desserts, salted snacks made from potatoes or cereals, food supplements, cosmetics. Could be carcinogenic.

In animal tests, this substance has caused genetic alterations and cancer.

- **E 131, Patent Blue V**, dye, carcinogenic? Permitted for: edible coatings for cheese and sausage (quantum satis), sweets (max. 300 mg/kg), cakes, cookies, puff pastries (max. 200 mg/kg), ice cream, desserts (max. 150 mg/kg), spirits, fruit wines (max. 200 mg/kg), cancer risk. Banned in the USA, Australia and Norway.
- **E 132 Indigo Carmine (Indigotine)**, hazardous colorant, may only be used for certain foods. These include: Confectionery (max. 300 mg/kg), cakes, cookies, puff pastry (max. 200 mg/kg), liqueur (max. 200 mg/l). Feeding experiments on mice showed evidence that indigotine in the presence of sodium nitrite becomes nitrosamines and these are carcinogenic.
- **E 133 Brilliant Blue FCF**, colorant, hazardous and approved only for certain products: edible coatings for cheese and sausage, sweets, pastries, wine spirits, ice cream.
- **E 142 Green S,** colorant, but only little used in Germany. Approved for: Confectionery (max. 200 mg/kg) Ice cream and desserts (max. 150 mg/kg) and for coloring pharmaceuticals, cosmetics and textiles. Banned in Canada, Japan, USA, Norway.
- **E 151 Brilliant Black BN**, colorant, very dangerous and may only be used in certain foods and in precisely defined quantities. Approved for: Seasoning sauces, confectionery (max. 300 mg/kg), meat and fish substitutes made from vegetable protein (max. 100 mg/kg), raw fish products (max. 300 mg/kg). Carcinogens. Banned in Finland, Canada, the USA, Japan and Norway.

- **E 154 Brown FK**, colorant, Brown FK is approved exclusively for "kippers" (smoked herring) (max. 20 mg/kg). It is used only very rarely. Suspected of being carcinogenic and banned in the USA.
- **E 155 Brown HT**, colorant, hazardous. Mainly used for confectionery. In feeding experiments, high doses of Brown HT were found to cause deposits in kidneys and lymphatics. Suspected of causing cancer.
- **E 160a, Beta Carotene**, ingestion of large amounts of this additive can cause lung cancer in smokers.
- **E 320 Butylated Hydroxyanisole** and **E321 Butylated Hydroxytoluene**, approved for cake mixes (max. 200 mg/kg), snack products from cereals (max. 200 mg/kg), dry soups and seasonings (max. 200 mg/kg), chewing gum. Research is still being conducted to determine whether they are carcinogenic.
- **E 249 Potassium Nitrite** and **E 250 Sodium Nitrite**, preservatives made from nitrates and nitrites, form so-called nitrosamines in interaction with protein building blocks (amines). They are among the most carcinogenic substances and have been shown to be harmful to the liver and genetic material in animal experiments.
- **E 951 sweetener Aspartame** is suspected of being involved in the development of cancer.
- **E 952 sweetener Cyclamate** has been banned in the USA since 1969. The sweetener is carcinogenic.
- **E 954 Saccharin**, feeding experiments in rats suggest a link with the development of bladder cancer.

- **E 330 Citric Acid**, antioxidant, complexing agent, acidifier, acidity regulator, melting salt. Approved for: Soft drinks (quantum satis), confectionery (qs), jam, marmalade, jelly (qs), ice cream and desserts (qs), fruit juices and fruit nectars (max. 3 or 5 g/l), sliced packaged vegetables, fruit and peeled potatoes (qs), cheese and meat products (qs), pasta. Citric acid is also used as a technical additive in the production of edible fats and the treatment of fresh fish.
  There are always warnings about it, because citric acid is produced in masses industrially by a mold. 1.4 million tons of citric acid are produced worldwide every year. This corresponds to more than ten times the acid content of the entire world lemon harvest. And a subspecies of this fungus actually produces highly carcinogenic substances.

qs = quantum satis (literally: sufficient quantity). A maximum quantity is not prescribed. However, only as much may be used as is necessary for the desired effect.

- **E210 Benzoic Acid**, very dangerous preservative. Permitted for: non-alcoholic beer in barrels, spirits (max. 200 mg/kg), sugar-reduced jams, marmalades, jellies (max. 500 mg/kg), olives (max. 500 mg/kg), egg paints. When combined with sorbic acid, approved for: candied or glazed fruits (max. 1,000 mg/kg), vegetables preserved in vinegar, oil or brine (max. 2,000 mg/kg), canned fish, dried fish and other fish products (200-2,000 mg/kg), shrimp (max. 6,000 mg/kg), chewing gum (max. 1,000 mg/kg), dietary foods for the obese (max. 1,500 mg/kg). Benzoic acid is also used in cosmetics and medicinal ointments. Benzoin pollutes the blood and has a link to leukemia in animals, as in humans, and is carcinogenic. Can damage the "procreative apparatus".

- **E 231, Orthophenyl Phenol**, preservative. Is approved for the treatment of citrus fruit surfaces only. Causes cancer in laboratory animals. Banned in Australia and the USA.
- **E236 Formic Acid**, preservative, carcinogenic. Approved for: Provolone cheese. Dangerous, banned in France.
- **E 239 Hexamethylene Tetramine**, preservative, is effective against bacteria, but hardly against yeasts and molds. However, it is not the substance itself that is effective, but formaldehyde. Formaldehyde itself is considered carcinogenic and may therefore no longer be used as a preservative in cosmetics. Hexamethylene tramine is only permitted for Provolone cheese. The maximum permissible value of 25 mg/kg refers to free formaldehyde.
- **E 241** and **E 240 Boric Acid,** preservative, authorized exclusively for real caviar. Maximum quantity restriction of 4 g/kg. Banned in France.
- **E 252 Potassium Nitrate** and **E 250 Sodium Nitrite**, hazardous preservatives, curing agents, curing salt. Approved for: cured meat products, cured pancetta, goose and duck liver pâté (also canned), hard and sliced cheese, pickled herring and sprats, but also for weapons and explosives. The substance is carcinogenic. In interaction with protein building blocks, the so-called nitrosamines are formed, which are very strong carcinogens. There is always a hard discussion whether the consumption of cured meat products is connected with cancers of the intestine and brain. Since this connection has not been disproved either, caution is advised.

I can't list all the E-numbers of concern here, but the above are the most common ones suspected of causing cancer.

On my website, www.dantse.dantse.com, "Anhang A" (Appendix A) is the entire list of approved additives (E-NUMBERS) in EU foods with properties, dosages and cancer hazard level (source Wikipedia). It is sorted by:

- Dyes, these make food look better,
- Preservatives, these increase the shelf life of food by delaying spoilage by molds or bacteria
- Antioxidants, they are intended to prevent quality loss due to reaction with atmospheric oxygen or other oxidizing chemicals
- Sweeteners, they are substitutes for sugar with a much stronger sweetening power
- Emulsifiers, stabilizers, thickeners and gelling agents. These excipients ensure the composition and structure of food preparations and conventional products or are required in the manufacturing process
- Anti-caking agents, acidity regulators. Anti-caking agents are release agents to prevent lumping at the consumer. Acidity regulators keep the desired pH value of a foodstuff constant
- Flavor enhancers, these enhance the taste and/or odor of a food product
- Other substances and substances without E-number

B7.2 Table of toxic and carcinogenic chemicals in foods

Poison	Occurrence	Explanation
Acrylamide	Chips, French fries, speculoos	Mutagenic, liver-damaging, probably carcinogenic. Acrylamide is also converted in the liver to the far more dangerous glycidamide
Agaritine	Raw mushrooms, dried mushrooms	Carcinogenic
Alcohol (ethanol)	Beer, wine, high-proof alcohols	Carcinogenic. Liver-damaging in large quantities. Highly addictive.
Anthraquinone	Partly contained in black tea. Partly in very questionable quantities.	Carcinogenic substance possibly formed during production process. Unresolved.
Antibiotics	Meat, seafood from aquaculture, dairy products	Promotes resistance to antibiotics and the emergence of super-resistant bacteria
Aluminum	Naturally present in many foods or via canned foods and aluminum kitchen utensils. Elevated levels in pretzels, tea.	Damages the brain. Possibly responsible for Alzheimer's disease

B7 Carcinogenic chemicals and toxins in food, households, agriculture

Poison	Occurrence	Explanation
Arsenic	Seaweed, fish, especially maties, seafood, especially mussels, rice, especially wholemeal and parboiled rice	May cause skin cancer, liver cancer with regular intake
Aspatarme	Sugar substitutes, sweets, diet products	May contain toxic impurities. Always contains toxic methanol. Suspected to be carcinogenic. E-number: E-951
Azo dyes	Candy, brightly colored food	Very questionable, carcinogenic dyes. Partly they contain: Benzidine. E numbers: E 102, E 104 (quinoline yellow), E 123, E 129, E 180
BHT	Desserts, chewing gum	Interferes with blood clotting, suspected cancer, may cause allergies. E number: E 321
Benzene	Partly in soft drinks, various food products	Benzene is carcinogenic. Can be formed if ascorbic acid or vitamin C is present in the beverage in addition to benzoic acid.

Poison	Occurrence	Explanation
Benzoic acid / sodium benzoate	Preservative. Naturally present in berries, blueberries, mushrooms. Extends shelf life of food. Partly contained in soft drinks.	Carcinogenic, can cause ADHD, headaches, digestive problems, allergy. In combination with ascorbic acid: can produce carcinogenic benzene.
Bisphenol A (BPA)	Plastic food packaging, plastic kettles (!), partly thermal paper, plastic kitchen containers, house dust, food cans.	Acts like hormone. Has a negative effect on fertility. May cause ADHD. Suspected cancer!
Cadmium	Dark chocolate, nuts, spinach, celery	Carcinogenic, nerve damaging, bone damaging. Originates from the natural composition of cultivated soils.
Cholesterol	In animal fats, especially in pork	Excessive intake promotes arteriosclerosis, increases risk of heart attack and stroke
Coumarin	Cinnamon cookies, woodruff	Harmful to liver, carcinogenic.
Cyclamate	Sugar substitute in diet products, sweets	Unresolved suspicion of causing cancer
Fungicides	Especially on citrus	Shall prevent fungal

B7 Carcinogenic chemicals and toxins in food, households, agriculture

Poison	Occurrence	Explanation
	fruits & strawberries	infestation of food.
Hardened fats	Margarine, convenience products, sweets, etc.	Accumulate in fatty tissue and are not broken down
Genetically modified food	Many vegetables and cereals affected. Must be declared in the EU if over 1% in food. No declaration requirement for animal feed for meat/dairy products.	Partly contain excessive pesticide load or unknown poisons. Impairs ecological agriculture, promotes patents on living beings!
Saturated fatty acids	Especially in animal fats, coconut fat	Have an unfavorable effect on cholesterol levels. Increased risk of heart attack and stroke.
Glutamate / flavor enhancer	Ready meals, snacks, Chinese dishes, yeast extract. Also occurs naturally in vegetables.	May cause intolerance in some people. Mild neurotoxin. E number: E 621
Glycidamide	French fries, potato chips, highly heated foods.	Formed during the digestion of acrylamide. Highly carcinogenic and mutagenic. Amounts in food are small.
Glyphosate	Widely used active ingredient in many	Most important chemical herbicide (weed control).

Poison	Occurrence	Explanation
	pesticides for "crop protection".	One of the brand names is "Roundup".
Histamine	In red wine, alcoholic beverages, canned fish (especially tuna), in cheese (the older, the more), sausage/ham and sauerkraut.	Is a toxic substance, does not need to be declared. May cause headaches and "hangover". Harmful to blood and heart. Very problematic for histamine allergy sufferers.
Melamine	Plastic, which is often used to make tableware.	By heating melamine tableware (from 70°C), melamine and formaldehyde get into the food. Risk of cancer and kidney disease.
Methanol	Main component of so-called fusel oils in alcohol. Partly also in fruit juices	Damages the nervous system. May cause blindness in higher doses. Toxic.
Mineral oil (MOSH / MOAH)	In various foods, e.g. edible oils, chocolate. Also through "staining" of cardboard recycling packaging and printing inks.	Mineral oil is harmful to health (including liver damage). However, due to contamination in the soil, during processing, through the packaging cannot always be avoided.

B7 Carcinogenic chemicals and toxins in food, households, agriculture

Poison	**Occurrence**	**Explanation**
Sodium nitrite, nitrite curing salt	In heated and then warm stored spinach, in highly heated cheese/sausage, and in cured foods.	E numbers: E 249; E 250; E 251; E 252. preservative. Other names for comparable substances: potassium nitrite, nitrate, potassium nitrate. Inhibits oxygen uptake of the blood.
Sodium fluoride Fluorine	In table salt, in Anglo-Saxon countries partly also added to tap water.	Is very toxic. Supposedly of essential importance for dental health.
Natamycin	Antibiotic-like substance in the rind of conventionally produced cheese. E 235.	May co-induce antibiotic resistance.
Nitrate	In drinking water, in various vegetables such as spinach, lettuce (in winter), chard and arugula (in winter).	Can be converted to carcinogenic nitrosamine in the stomach.
Patent blue	In food as a blue color.	Rather harmless. May cause allergies.

Poison	Occurrence	Explanation
PET bottles: Acetaldehyde/ Estrogen	PET bottles are often used as packaging for beverages.	Acetaldehyde, which is harmful to the liver and cells, is released from the plastic into the beverage. In addition, estrogen-like hormones are often found in the contents of the bottles.
Phthalates	Plastic food packaging	Phthalates dissolve through fat or liquids and pass into food. They are found, for example, in soft films around sliced cheese or in coatings on food cans.
Phytoestrogen	Soy / tofu products, beans	Hormone-like effect, cancer-promoting in some women at extremely high levels of consumption.
Polycyclic hydrocarbons (PAH)	Grilled and smoked foods	Formed during incomplete combustion and are carcinogenic. Partly contained in black teas.

B7 Carcinogenic chemicals and toxins in food, households, agriculture

Poison	Occurrence	Explanation
Pyrrolizidine alkaloids	Occurs partly in herbal teas (especially chamomile, lemon balm) and honey, and in arugula.	Is a natural component of plants toxic to humans. Extremely toxic substance!
Radioactivity	Occurrence in food: Wild meat, wild mushrooms, goods from contaminated areas (e.g. Fukushima, or Pacific). Also due to uranium partly in mineral waters.	Beware of wild mushrooms, seaweed, tuna.
Saccharin	Sugar substitutes, sweets, diet products	Unresolved suspicion of causing cancer in large quantities.
Safrole	Nutmeg, camphor, rootberry	Toxic
Mold toxin / Aflatoxins etc.	Cereals, bread, pistachios, peanuts, coffee, tomatoes tarnished brown (blight).	Harmful to liver, carcinogenic

Poison	Occurrence	Explanation
Melting salts, phosphates	Processed cheese, cheeseburger etc. E 450 to E 495 (sodium phosphates, potassium phosphate, calcium phosphate etc.)	Damages kidneys, destabilizes bones, overall harmful effect. Life-threatening for kidney patients.
Semicarbazide	Plastic coated lids of beverages and food jars	Harmful to health. Acts like a hormone.
Silicones	Silicone additives in frying oil, especially in fast food chains. Name: E 900	The silicone itself is not toxic (although of concern because it is petroleum-based), but it multiplies acrylamide levels in fried products.
Solanine	Poison in the stem of the tomato, in unripe tomatoes, in potato shoots.	Weak Poison.
Stevia	Sweet drinks and sweets	Considered relatively harmless if not eaten too much. Maximum amount: 2g /day.
Sulfites	Wine, spirits, dried fruit, potato products	Health concern. Sodium disulfite destroys vitamin B1 in the body. Also problematic for allergy sufferers.

B7 Carcinogenic chemicals and toxins in food, households, agriculture

Poison	Occurrence	Explanation
Trans fatty acids	Microwave popcorn, fried baked goods, puff pastry, French fries, potato chips, cookies (especially in products with "hydrogenated fats").	Harmful to health. See saturated fatty acids.
Vanillin	Confectionery, ready meals, in tobacco products	Artificial vanilla flavoring. Slightly harmful to health. Carcinogenic in large quantities or when burned.
Caramel coloring (ammonium sulfite)	Coke, drinks, sweets, whisky, jams	Sulfite ammonium caramel (E 150d) is contained in cola and is considered problematic. Inducing convulsions in animal experiments. Contains the carcinogenic substance 4-methylimidazole.

This is only an excerpt. (Source: http://www.gesundheitstabelle.e/index.php/schadstoffe-gifte/gifte-kosmetika)

B7.3 Carcinogenic heavy metals in food

Nitrite, nitrate

It has been known since 1969 that nitrite (for example E 252, E 251) is present in foods, especially in meat, cheese and fish, which can lead to nitrosamine reactions in the stomach. Many pharmaceuticals form nitrosamine compounds with nitrite from food as well, which are extremely effective carcinogens.

Dioxins and the dioxin-like polychlorinated biphenyls (PCBs).

These chlorine-containing substances are very toxic, some even carcinogenic. More than 80% of the total intake comes from food such as meat, fish, eggs or milk, where the maximum limit is regularly exceeded. The cases are often not even known. Or only when it is too late and the contaminated products are already on the market and consumed. Dioxins are colorless and odorless organic compounds containing carbon, hydrogen, oxygen and chlorine. According to Wikipedia, PCBs are toxic and carcinogenic organic chlorine compounds that were used until the 1980s primarily in transformers, electrical capacitors, in hydraulic systems as hydraulic fluids, and as plasticizers in paints, sealants, insulants and plastics. Like dioxins, PCBs are fat-loving and, in some cases, very persistent. They accumulate in the fatty tissue of humans and animals. Because dioxins and PCBs love fat, the risk of ingesting these substances increases with the fat content of food. Dioxins and PCBs are very long-lived substances. They hardly break down once they are stored in fatty tissue. The older you get and with continuous intake of the toxins, the higher the level in your body increases and this also means a higher chance of developing cancer.

The most dangerous carcinogenic heavy metals that can be found in food are lead, cadmium and mercury.

Lead accumulates in bones and teeth and is particularly damaging to the nervous system and the hematopoietic system. In animal experiments, lead has also caused cancer.

Cadmium is preferentially stored in the kidneys, but also in other organs such as the liver, thyroid gland and bones. Especially in the vicinity of busy roads and industrial plants, the concentration and absorption of cadmium becomes very significant. Cadmium mainly causes lung cancer.

Mercury is mainly ingested through the consumption of fish and marine animals, mostly in the form of organic mercury compounds. Mercury compounds have shown carcinogenic effects in animal studies.

Arsenic used to be used in paints and pesticides, for example. Today it is found in the workplace. Arsenic can cause lung cancer, rarely skin cancer, and possibly other tumors, e.g. of the bladder.

Chromium, nickel and cobalt can also be carcinogenic in food.

B7.4 Carcinogens in milk and dairy products

"If your life were as bitter as mine, and you had to witness this massacre of innocent children by a totally inappropriate diet day after day, I think you would feel just as I do: This misguided propaganda about infant nutrition should be considered murder of children. Anyone who, through ignorance or even recklessness, causes a baby to be fed unsuitable food may be found guilty of the baby's death."-Dr. Cicely Williams, Milk and Murder, 1939. She was a prominent pediatrician and delivered this speech in

Singapore in 1939. (Translation: http://www.zentrum-der-gesundheit.de/babynahrung.html)

When I was a child, I asked my father why Africans didn't breed milk cows and why we didn't drink milk in the morning like the Europeans in the commercials, but ate something warm instead? We would have money enough for that, after all (drinking milk for breakfast and eating white bread at that time 40 years ago was only something for people who wanted to show that they could afford it. Milk was very expensive because it had to be imported from Europe. It was a way to show that you lived in prosperity and my father could have done that). He answered: "Because cow is cow and man is man. Our tradition does not invent anything that can harm man. Cow's milk is not healthy for humans. The milk seems to have certain good properties, but in traditional studies it was found that cow's milk can cause certain diseases in humans." Then he asked me, "Why should an adult human still drink milk? That would be unique in the world. Nature didn't intend it that way. Milk is there for children's growth, not for adult nutrition."

Another experience really gave me a wake-up call. I was already in Germany and my mother visited me. Every morning I ate cereal with plenty of milk, as was propagated everywhere. That is so healthy, gives strength, so I always bragged after exercising. One day my mother was in the kitchen, suddenly looked at me strangely and snidely and said, "Guy, do you really think what you're eating right now is healthy?" I was so amazed that she asked that. My mother, being from Africa, didn't go to college. How would she know what gives strength? All the scientific reports talk about milk as an all-healer and she comes and wants to tell me something, I thought arrogantly and confidently. Then she even went on with her warning, "The bone pain you talk about could even come from that and your constant bad breath comes from dairy products. Watch out, son! Milk does something to men's genitals. We've known for a long time that milk can cause diseases in the male reproductive organs and milk also weakens your manhood. If you've been failing in bed lately, lay off milk for a while and you'll see. Our problem is that in our culture we don't provide evidence because little is written." These yet very precise warnings from my mother really led me at that time to stop consuming milk and yogurt on a regular basis. In fact, those constant pains in my bones went away. My girlfriend complimented me at one point that my bad breath was gone. Then, when I really started to feel a lot more like it again in bed, I decided to do some research on milk and dairy products, and I've covered it quite a bit in my books.

Yes, that was my little "anecdote" about milk.

Is milk really a factor of cancer?

Before and during the writing of this book, as I mentioned at the beginning of the book, I was constantly doing surveys, constantly on forums, often chatting with people who suffered from cancer or people who had something to do with it. It struck me that the vast majority of women who had cancer had a high consumption of dairy products, especially cheese. They cooked a lot with cream and baked a lot with milk. Among women who did not have cancer, the vast majority ate little dairy and cheese. I know this is not a scientific study and is hard to generalize to the general public but for me, these findings were helpful.

As with pills, chemotherapy, radiation, and some drugs, opinions among scientists about dairy products are very different and highly controversial. Some think that because of the high calcium content, because of the proteins, fats and carbohydrates in an almost ideal ratio, milk and milk derivatives are excellent foods. But many studies warn that milk and milk products can also cause cancer. Milk contains high levels of estrogen and progesterone, which can significantly increase the risk of breast, ovarian and uterine cancer. Dairy cows' feed has very little to do with greens and all the more to do with concentrated feed, which is still diligently treated with chemicals and poisons (pesticides, herbicides, fungicides, drugs, etc.), critics say. Their criticism is fueled by the increasing prevalence of lactose intolerance in the population. Cow's milk is healthy for calves, and only during the time when they cannot yet eat grass. Nature did not intend for humans to still drink milk in adulthood, they stress.

Some studies show an increased risk of cancer from milk, others do not come to this conclusion. As always, opponents and proponents accuse each other of being conspiracy theorists, alarmists, barracudas, or scientists in the pay of business and capital.

It is clear that milk and products made from milk are staple foods in Western countries. Most dishes, pastries, cakes, chocolate, sweets, contain more or less something based on milk. That's why milk is essential for the economy and food industry and we consumers will end up not knowing exactly what is true and what is not. Also reports from the media can be tendentious because of this.

In the spirit of this book, I would like to present facts and information from my research that should lead consumers to broaden their view of milk and better assess risks.

Even if we assume that milk is healthy, the question would be whether the industrially processed cow's milk would also still be valuable? To make the milk durable, it is heated, filtered and processed (pasteurized or homogenized, etc.). The ingredients of the new milk have thus been altered and lose their effectiveness. The new milk has nothing to do with the natural milk anymore. The good fat, for example, is so finely filtered by these industrial processes that it is no longer as good for the human body as the original fat.

Now what does a serious scientific study from Harvard University say about this? It sees a connection between cancer and pasteurized (industrial) milk.

A group of researchers, led by doctor Ganmaa Davaasambuu, sees a link between pasteurized milk and cancer (breast cancer, prostate cancer, ovarian cancer), according to a study. Industrially processed milk in the USA was examined. Natural milk from Mongolia served as a comparative value. Hormone-dependent forms of cancer in particular, such as breast or prostate cancer (maybe my mother was right after all when she said that milk can cause problems in the genital area of men?) are said to be favored by industrial milk. In this study, industrial milk was found to contain 33 times more estrogen than natural milk from Mongolia. Doctor Davaasambuu told the *Harvard Gazette*, "The milk we drink today may have nothing to do with nature's perfect food."

The study suspects the cause in the type of feed and animal husbandry in modern farms. Hormones and drugs are added to the animals' feed and these end up in the milk. According to the Harvard study, there would be a possible link between the female sex hormones in the milk of pregnant cows and the development of breast, ovarian and uterine cancer. Previous cancer studies also pointed to milk consumption.

An international comparative study confirmed Dr. Davaasambuu's hypothesis that consumption of dairy products increases the likelihood of developing cancer. The relationship between dietary habits and cancer rates in 42 countries was studied. It was found that there was a relationship between dairy or cheese consumption and testicular cancer. Cancer rates were highest in countries like Switzerland, where a lot of cheese is consumed. In countries where dairy products are consumed little or rarely, fewer cases were reported.

A clear link between milk and cancer is also emerging in Japan. The number of cases of prostate cancer and breast cancer has risen sharply with increased milk consumption over the last 50 years.

Breast cancer studies again specifically warned against milk and cheese. Another study confirmed that rats fed milk were more likely to develop tumors than rats that drank water instead.

On the website of Harvard School of Public Health (http://www.hsph.harvard.edu/nutritionsource/what-should-you-eat/calcium-and-milk/)
it says: "...Calcium is important. But milk isn't the only, or even best, source... While calcium and dairy can lower the risk of osteoporosis and colon cancer, high intake can increase the risk of prostate cancer and possibly ovarian cancer."

A report on milk on the Bavarian television website also confirms the suspicions of a link between cancer and dairy products, although the report is very cautious:

"When is it healthy? When does it make you sick? ... At the moment, the study situation is that increased milk consumption can reduce the risk of colon cancer. Possibly, however, milk consumption increases the risk of prostate cancer. However, this is only the case if a lot of calcium is consumed at the same time as little vitamin D... In other words, you should never eat more than 1,500 mg of calcium per day and make sure that you get enough vitamin D. In the case of breast cancer, the studies are inconclusive..."

Nitrite compounds

It is known that nitrite is present in many cheeses and other dairy products, which can react in the stomach to form nitrosamines. Also, many pharmaceuticals form nitrosamine compounds with nitrite from food, which are extremely effective carcinogens.

Aflatoxin B1

An extremely dangerous carcinogenic substance in milk.

Aflatoxins are naturally occurring fungal toxins that were first identified in mold. There are over 20 naturally occurring aflatoxins, of which aflatoxin B1 is considered the most dangerous to humans. In addition to aflatoxin B1, the toxins B2, G1 and G2 and the derivatives M1 and M2, which occur in milk, are of particular importance.

"Aflatoxins have an acute hepatotoxic effect (liver dystrophy) at concentrations around 10 µg/kg body weight, but are carcinogenic to mammals, birds, and fish at lower concentrations and especially with repeated ingestion. The lethal dose of aflatoxin B1 in adults is 1 to 10 mg/kg body weight when ingested orally. In animal studies with rats (lethal dose 7.2 mg/kg body weight), the carcinogenicity of a daily dose of 10 µg/kg body weight was clearly demonstrated. Aflatoxin B1 is thus one of the most potent carcinogenic compounds of all." (Wikipedia)

Aflatoxins are heat-stable and are destroyed only to a small extent during cooking or baking. They can be ingested through food or contaminated air

If aflatoxin-containing agricultural products are fed as animal feed, the aflatoxins can pass into foodstuffs such as milk. Aflatoxin is a mold toxin that is highly carcinogenic when ingested over long periods.

Because of the dangerous effect of aflatoxins, limit values (maximum levels) have been set in many countries around the world and also within the European Union.

Dioxins and the dioxin-like polychlorinated biphenyls (PCBs)

These chlorine-containing substances are very toxic and some are even carcinogenic. They are found in milk and milk derivatives. Since dioxins and PCBs love fat, the risk for humans to ingest these substances increases with the fat content of the food. Dioxins and PCBs are very durable substances. They hardly break down once they are stored in fatty tissue. The older one gets, with continuous ingestion of the toxins, the higher the content in the body increases and this also means an increased risk of cancer.

Milk, osteoporosis and other ailments

In my research, I found old studies showing that milk could lead to osteoporosis. Dr. Ganmaa Davaasambuu comments, "In terms of estrogen exposure for humans, cow's milk worries us the most because it contains a significant amount of female sex hormones."

I know from my own experience what a reduction in milk and dairy consumption brings, and I also know that many people around me and many of my clients who have largely given up dairy products report feeling better (improvement in body odor and skin, disappearance of migraines, weight loss, especially around the hips and abdomen, disappearance of painful periods, strengthening of sexual desire and virility, etc.).

The continuing increase in the incidence of hormone-controlled cancers worldwide must compel us to also discuss intensively about the possible role of endogenous estrogens through diet! And it just so happens that cow's milk contains considerable amounts of estrogens.

This means that there are indications that should lead us humans to carefully examine our attitude towards milk. Maybe the ancient African wisdom is right after all? But I know that it will remain a tough argument about what milk can do and what milk can harm. The best thing to do is to give it up for a while to experience the changes in your own body and soul.

B7.5 Carcinogenic substances in breast milk

Toxins such as those from tobacco and alcohol consumption, hashish, other drugs and other highly toxic and carcinogenic substances rapidly pass into breast milk and poison the baby. Nicotine reaches a concentration in breast milk three times higher than in the mother's blood.

Carcinogenic substances in tea, coffee, coke and lemonade also end up very quickly in breast milk. Breastfeeding teas are sometimes heavily contaminated with harmful substances that could be carcinogenic, and some coffee contains the substance furan. This is suspected of promoting cancer.

The Federal Institute for Risk Assessment warned in summer 2013 that many herbal teas are contaminated with carcinogenic substances! Especially children, pregnant women and nursing mothers should not drink too much herbal tea.

All these toxins end up in the mother's milk very quickly and can thus harm the babies.

Dioxins and the dioxin-like polychlorinated biphenyls (PCBs) in breast milk

These chlorine-containing substances are very toxic and some are carcinogenic. Since they are present in food and love anything that is fatty, they can reach the baby through fatty breast milk even after eating products that contain these toxins. This is also true for other toxins, such as nitrosamines, dangerous preservatives, dyes, etc., which babies can absorb through breast milk.

It is therefore of great importance to pay attention to what you let in when you are pregnant or breastfeeding a baby.

7.6 Carcinogenic substances in baby food

Ökotest, a German consumer magazine, has found that certain baby foods are contaminated with carcinogenic substances. In "Hipp mashed potatoes with early carrots & tender organic beef", the testers even found a sometimes highly elevated benzene and furan content. Both substances are considered carcinogenic. Benzene is known as a component of gasoline, furan is used as a resin for molding materials. Benzene is clearly carcinogenic, while this is suspected in the case of furan on the basis of animal experiments.

Benzene was also found in "Sanostol," a juice used as a dietary supplement for children.

Sweeteners in children's foods

Sweeteners, such as saccharin, aspartame or cyclamate are popular with the industry because they are much cheaper than sugar. Aspartame is a dangerous sweetener that is carcinogenic. Many scientific studies prove this. However, the critical studies about it are underrated. Neotame E 961 is also a sweetener of the aspartame kind but even sweeter. In my research, some children's foods seemed to contain the substance, but it is not always required to be labeled everywhere. Many critics rate neotame as even more toxic than aspartame.

E 473 is the additive sugar ester of fatty acids, which is suspected of causing cancer and is unfortunately found in baby foods.

Baby foods can also be poisoned by external substances. For example

- by silicone pacifiers containing PAH compounds-naphthalene (Ökotest August 2012). PAH is an abbreviation for polycyclic aromatic hydrocarbons and they are suspected of being carcinogenic.
- Bisphenol in baby bottles is very dangerous because bisphenol is suspected of causing cancer. Bisphenol A (BPA) is a chemical compound used mainly in combination with other chemical substances in the production of plastics and resins. For example, BPA is used in polycarbonate, a transparent, rigid, high-performance plastic; polycarbonate, in

turn, is used to make food containers such as reusable beverage bottles, baby bottles. The Canadian government was the first to ban bisphenol A (BPA) in baby bottles in 2008. Bisphenol dissolves out of plastic when heated in microwave or kettle and generally boiling water!

In Part B Chapter 7.4. "Carcinogenic substances in milk and dairy products" I also reported how children can ingest dangerous carcinogenic substances through cow's milk and cow's milk products. Even the baby's best food, breast milk, can be poisoned, see the previous chapter 7.5.

B7.7 Carcinogens in meat and meat products

In 2009, a large-scale study was presented by the U.S. National Institute often Health (NIH) and it said, "People who eat a lot of meat from cattle, pigs and lambs, or sausage made from them, have a significantly higher risk of dying from cancer or heart attack than someone who eats little or hardly any meat."

In my opinion, it is not due to the meat directly. It's the same with industrial and natural cow's milk. In Cameroon, for example, people eat a lot of beef, especially the people in northern Cameroon. If it were only the pure meat, they and also the entire population of the neighboring country Chad would have to be ill with cancer, because they live almost exclusively on meat. Meat makes up more than 50% of the meals there. We are talking about kilos of meat per week per person. No, said one researcher I approached about it, it's because of the toxins we put on the animals and the toxins we use for processing. Through heating and other processes, they interact and dangerous chemicals like nitrosamines (HHA) and hydrocarbons (PAHs) can emerge. They are suspected of causing cancer. After the animals have been pumped full of growth hormones, antibiotics, drugs and genetically "tailored" feed, and the meat has been treated with all kinds of chemicals during further processing, it goes without saying that eating meat can also make you really sick.

That it is the chemicals in the animals that make the meat dangerous can also be read in the book "Chemicals in Foodstuffs", published by the Katalyse-Umweltgruppe Köln ev. Animals are injected with artificial hormones (which are substances that act like estrogen but are not chemically related to it at all) to reduce feed consumption and achieve rapid growth. One such hormone is called diethylstilbestrol (DES), which is used to treat calves illicitly. Residues of DES in meat can lead to more serious diseases. Treatment of pregnant women with the synthetic hormone led to vaginal cancer in their daughters.

Many hormones used on animal farms were not subject to environmental assessment when they were approved for marketing. In humans, an increase in hormone-dependent cancers has been observed for several years. Fertility problems in men and women and an increasingly early onset of puberty have also been observed.

Steroids are very dangerous and are used in feedlots. These drugs, which are considered to be genetically harmful and carcinogenic, are used, among other things, in sow husbandry for cycle equalization.

In general terms, hormonally active substances can be associated with, among other things, disorders in organ development, reduction in male fertility and increased incidence of certain forms of cancer. To the detriment of consumers, all data on hormones used in livestock production and their amounts are not open.

Meat products such as sausage, salami, canned foods, etc. are also often processed with hazardous chemicals (see the tables on hazardous additives in food in Part A. Of course, this is how these chemicals get into us and can cause cancer). Preservatives, such as sodium nitrite and sodium nitrate, are used to preserve the products, which increase the risk of cancer. The carcinogenic nitrosamines are produced by baking a pizza with salami or grilling cured meat.

The *Daily Mail* quotes a study according to which researchers in Sweden found that eating as little as 50 grams of processed meat such as salami daily increases the likelihood of developing cancer by 19 percent and eating 150 grams daily increases it by as much as 57 percent.

Cured meat and sausage is meat that has been processed by preservatives. During the curing process, the use of the nitrate or nitrite causes the so-called reddening. Studies have confirmed a link between the intake of nitrite from cured meats and sausages and certain types of cancer. Cured meat can cause cancer. A frequent diet of foods containing nitrite or nitrite-cured salt, such as ham or sausage, increases the risk of developing cancer, according to one study.

The German Cancer Research Center assumes that the registered decrease in stomach cancer cases is due to the reduced use of cured or smoked foods (Wikipedia).

Some antibiotics, such as chloramphenicol, which are used against bacterial infections in animals - in pigs, cattle and chickens - are carcinogenic. There used to be furazolidone, dimetridazole, chloramphenicol, for example, which were banned in the 1990s but were still used for a long time. "There are a number of veterinarians and farmers who don't give a damn about official bans and who pump their animals full of substances that may yet harm humans," to quote the *Berliner Zeitung.*

More and more often we hear about contaminated animal feed by dioxins and the dioxin-like polychlorinated biphenyls (PCBs). These chlorine-containing substances are very toxic and some are carcinogenic. They poison not only the meat, but also the milk of the animals and the drinking water. Thus, they very easily get into the human body and become a danger for it, because dioxin is a very strong carcinogenic substance.

Heavy metals such as cadmium, lead or arsenic in meat can also be harmful to health. They enter the animals mainly via feed (fish meal, grain, grass, etc.). The animals are also sometimes heavily contaminated with heavy metals via the air they breathe, and these then enter humans when they eat meat.

B7.8 Carcinogens in fish

Many people switch to fish and therefore believe they are eating something healthier than meat. Unfortunately, many consumers do not know that there are also dangerous substances in fish. Most of the fish we get on the market are farmed fish and they are treated and fed with chemicals of all kinds just like other farmed/cultured animals. Researchers are discovering more and more toxins in food fish from aquaculture. Some of them are carcinogenic.

This is the case, for example, with malachite green. This protects fish from fungal infections and parasites. Although the agent is banned, breeders manage to use it again and again. However, it is suspected of causing cancer.

Salmon farming has a bad reputation: the animals get poor feed and are treated with antibiotics. An American researcher has now discovered that salmon meat is additionally contaminated with carcinogenic chemicals.

Food chemists at the University of Stuttgart-Hohenheim found elevated levels of potentially carcinogenic substances in food fish in 2007. They found elevated concentrations of dangerous natural substances in the fat of lake fish from aqua farms. These are very similar to the carcinogenic polybrominated organic substances previously used as flame retardants in fittings or computer housings.

But not only farmed fish can be dangerous for humans, fish from nature can carry dangerous toxins too, due to environmental and water pollution (seas, lakes, rivers) by illegal or legal disposal (waste oil, chemicals). It has been proven that residues of agricultural chemicals, painkillers and birth control pills are increasingly found in our rivers. The Austrian Board of Trustees for Fisheries and Water Protection (ÖKF) drew attention in a press release to the fact that about 100,000 chemicals enter wastewater every day (cleaning agents, disinfectants, cosmetics, products from veterinary and human medicine, e.g. birth control pill, pesticides and weed killers, plasticizers and flame retardants from the plastics industry). Since most sewage treatment plants are not yet able to filter these substances out of wastewater, they enter water bodies and are ingested by fish and also pollute drinking water. Thus, these carcinogenic toxins enter the food chain and ultimately humans. Studies have shown in animal experiments that the combination of different substances can be carcinogenic. They damaged the genetic material and, as *EU research*, the scientific journal of the European Union, wrote: "These substances can cause feminization of aquatic life and even locally the disappearance of certain species". One can imagine what this could cause in humans.

Canned fish is sometimes treated with nitrate (No.3) as a preservative. During storage, part of the nitrate is transformed into nitrite (No.2) and the nitrite together with amines of the fish forms nitrosamines. Nitrosamines are very strong carcinogens.

Smoking fish and meat products can produce substances that have been shown to be carcinogenic in animal experiments. These are so-called polycyclic aromatic hydrocarbons - PAHs, which are formed during the combustion of organic materials.

Dioxins and the dioxin-like polychlorinated biphenyls (PCBs): These chlorine-containing substances are very toxic and some are carcinogenic. They are also present in fish.

Mercury levels in fish

Higher levels of toxins, such as dioxins, PCBs (polychlorinated biphenyls) and mercury above the tolerated limit are found in some fish. Scientists agree that methylmercury is an extremely dangerous substance. All of these chemicals are carcinogenic if the maximum limit is exceeded.

Other heavy metals in fish are cadmium, arsenic, lead.

B7.9 Carcinogens in poultry meat and poultry products, duck, chicken, chicken nuggets, eggs

The same applies to poultry and poultry products as described in Part B, Chapter 7.7 "Carcinogenic substances in meat and meat products".

B7.10 Carcinogens in cereals (flour, rice, soy, corn, wheat, etc.), bread, refined flour

Cereals can also contain carcinogenic toxins, such as glyphosate. In agriculture, however, the world's most widely sold herbicide is readily used to make grain harvesting easier. The plant poison is suspected of damaging the genetic makeup of humans and animals and causing diseases such as cancer.

According to investigations by BUND and ÖKO-TEST, the herbicide was detected in the urine of 182 metropolitans from 18 European countries. 70 percent of all samples in Germany were contaminated. Seven out of ten metropolitans in Germany tested had the herbicide in their urine, according to BUND. This is proof that - contrary to the promises of the producers - this active ingredient is spreading through the food chain and the population in Europe is largely contaminated with glyphosate.

In 2012, ÖKO-TEST had flour, oatmeal and baked goods tested for glyphosate and found it in 14 of 20 samples. Most notably, eight of the ten rolls tested were contaminated, proving that glyphosate survives baking temperatures.

Jürgen Stellpflug, editor-in-chief of ÖKO-TEST says:

"Our test results show that glyphosate is getting into people's bodies through food. Glyphosate does not belong in food, pesticides do not belong in the human body. What's appalling is the failure of regulators to do much testing for such exposures to glyphosate, of all things, the most widely used pesticide in the world."

Refined flour can also be dangerous. A study published in the journal *Cancer Epidemiology, Mile Markers, and Prevention* found that regular consumption of refined carbohydrates can increase breast cancer in women by 22%. All high-glycemic foods (cereals, bread and baked goods, cake, crackers and chips, candy) are known to increase blood sugar levels in the body very quickly, and this promotes the growth and spread of cancer cells.

The highly carcinogenic aflatoxin B1 is also present in some cereals such as corn, wheat and rice.

B7.11 Carcinogens in French fries, potato chips, popcorn, donuts, hot dogs

French fries, chips and the like contain dangerous carcinogenic substances.

French fries

In French fries and potato chips, scientists from the Technical University of Munich have detected a substance that is "significantly more dangerous" than acrylamide - the carcinogenic **glycidamide!** Glycidamide is significantly more dangerous than acrylamide, which was discovered in potato products years ago. It is considered to be highly carcinogenic. Even the smallest amounts could elicit mutations.

Acrylamide is also formed during frying and was first detected in high quantities in food in 2002, according to the Federal Institute for Risk Assessment. In animal studies, acrylamide was carcinogenic.

Trans fatty acids in French fries can also be carcinogenic. Similar to donuts, French fries are deep-fried. Most fast food chains use hydrogenated fat. Trans fats thus end up in the fries or even in chicken wings. The risk of cancer increases. Trans fatty acids are formed during the industrial hardening of oils, such as in the production of margarines, baking or spreadable fats, but also during intense heating, such as deep-frying. Chemically hardened oils are popular with industry: they can be heated at a very high temperature, they last longer and they are cheaper. Many countries have already banned trans fats or reduced their consumption. Trans fats not only increase the risk of cancer, but they are also responsible for many other diseases. They can even harm unborn children.

If the body takes in trans fats, they settle where unsaturated fatty acids (in nuts, fish) were intended. The trans fats replace the unsaturated fat purely physically, but they cannot fulfill the functions of the unsaturated fatty acids (such as cell function of the brain, glandular function, oxygen transport). This leads to misunderstanding and impairment in the body, which ultimately causes harm.

The consumption of trans fats has a negative effect on the feeling of hunger. People who eat a lot of foods that contain trans fats feel that they are not quite full. This is because the body is not getting the fatty acids it needs. This leads to eating more, and that in turn leads to weight gain. And obesity is one of the conditions that promotes cancer. Especially belly fat promotes the development of cancer.

Chips, crackers, cookies, crispbread and fried onions should also be enjoyed with caution. In addition to sugar, these also contain trans fats, as in French fries and donuts. Unfortunately, trans fats are not listed on packaging, which would greatly protect consumers. Trans fats only have to be listed if the food contains more than 0.5 grams per serving, according to naturalnews.com. To avoid listing, manufacturers reduce the amounts listed until the trans fatty acid value is less than 0.5 grams.

Furthermore, white refined flour is used in the production of chips and cookies. This flour, like large amounts of sugar, is also harmful and promotes cancer.

Donuts

I have already written about a clear link between cancer risk and trans fats in French fries. Trans fats are used in the production of donuts. When hydrogenated fat is heated, artificial trans fats are created. Thus, there are vegetable oils that are hydrogenated to have a longer shelf life, their consumption increases the risk of cancer.

Popcorn

Microwave popcorn is convenient but can be dangerous: As Canadian chemists have now discovered, phosphate esters (PAPs), often found in fast food packaging and microwave popcorn, enter the human body where they are degraded to perfluorinated carboxylic acids (PDCAs). These substances are detectable in humans worldwide and are strongly suspected of being a possible elicitor for cancer.

Hot Dogs

Children should eat no more than 12 hot dogs per month, recommends the U.S. Cancer Prevention Coalition, according to naturalnews.com. That's because hot dogs contain so-called nitrates. These are often added to meat to make it more durable. Nitrates also make meat and sausage appear pink rather than brown. The nitrate can turn into nitrite when heated. Nitrite and amines (proteins) are involved in the formation of nitrosamines in the body. Nitrosamines are carcinogenic (stomach cancer).

B7.12 Carcinogens in vegetables, edible mushrooms, fruit

Fruits and vegetables are healthy: You should eat plenty of fruits and vegetables every day, experts recommend. But fruits and vegetables from conventional cultivation can actually harm health, because they can contain carcinogenic pesticides. In addition, cadmium and lead can be found in vegetables and grains. Tofu sausages also contain pesticides and plasticizers. In general, as one expert told me, eating vegetarian products does not make you less harmful, you just collect other harmful substances.

Pesticides have long been suspected of having a possible carcinogenic effect. This has been denied time and again. But studies and observations show that pesticides can cause cancer. In Argentina, where the pesticide active ingredient glyphosate, which is actually considered "relatively harmless," is used together with genetically modified soy plants, a sharp increase in cancer cases has been found in the vicinity of the cultivation areas. More malformations and genetic damage in newborns and chronic diseases have also been recorded. In early 2011, the use of pesticides near settlements was completely banned in the region.

B7 Carcinogenic chemicals and toxins in food, households, agriculture

Several pesticides are known to have hormonal effects that can lead to fertility problems, prostate and breast cancer. This effect can be triggered by even very small doses. There is evidence of endocrine disruption in over 40 pesticides used in Europe, and residues of over 30 of them have been detected in food. In 2012, Global 2000, an Austrian environmental protection organization, presented a study on hormonally active pesticides in European fruit and vegetables.

"The average levels of endocrine disrupting pesticides determined for the five varieties mentioned range from 600 micrograms per kilogram (apples, leeks) to 1,300 micrograms per kilogram (green lettuce). By comparison, a birth control pill contains a maximum of 200 micrograms of synthetic estrogen and progestin hormones. This is worrying," said Helmut Burtscher, environmental chemist at Global 2000.

Together with the "Pesticide Action Network", they had evaluated the monitoring data of the European Food Authority from 27 EU member states. The results were clear: there is a high level of exposure to pesticides containing chemicals that interfere with hormone balance. Particularly affected are lettuce, tomatoes, cucumbers, apples, grapes, leeks.

Residues of prochloraz can be found in various foods. Apples, peppers and strawberries are most affected, but residues can also be found in beans, cauliflower, mandarins and oranges (EFSA, 2009). Prochloraz is very dangerous (feminization of male offspring as well as malformations of the sexual organs, thyroid hormone disorders). Despite the alarming evidence from scientific studies, prochloraz is approved as a pesticide for the European market and is often used in conventional agriculture in Germany and in Austria, e.g. in arable farming.

In addition, the American researchers suspect an influence of pesticides (including prochloraz) on brain development. Accordingly, children whose mothers had eaten fruits and vegetables contaminated with so-called organic phosphates during pregnancy later have a lower intelligence quotient.

B7.13 Top 10 most hormonally contaminated fruits and vegetables and top 10 most common hormonal pesticide residues

(Source: Global 2000, as of 2008)

1	2	3
Lettuce	**Tomatoes**	**Cucumbers**
1. dithiocarbamates*	1. dithiocarbamates*	1. dithiocarbamates*
2. iprodione	2. captan	2. propamocarb
3. propamocarb	3. iprodione	3. iprodione
4. cypermethrin	4. chlorothalonil	4. chlorothalonil
5. deltamethrin	5. deltamethrin	5. deltamethrin
6. tolclofosmethyl	6. flutriazole	6. cypermethrin
7. chlorothalonil	7. cypermethrin	7. myclobutanil
8. bifenthrin	8. myclobutanil	8. cyproconazole
9. pirimicarb	9. pyrimethanil	9. tebuconazole
10. methomyl	10. propamocarb	10. penconazole

4	5	6	7	8	9	10

Apple	Leek	Nectarine	Strawberr y	Pear	Grape	Pepper

Fruits and vegetables with the lowest amount of EDC (Endocrine Disrupting Chemicals).

1	2	3	4	5
Carrot	**Spinach**	**Potato**	**Pea**	**Banana**

B7.14 Carcinogenic substances in dry Fruits and nuts

Aflotoxins are metabolic products of molds. Aflatoxins can occur due to pre- or post-harvest fungal infestation in peanuts, tree nuts, corn, rice, figs and other dried fruits, spices, raw vegetable oils and cocoa beans. Aflotoxin B1 is among the most potent carcinogens of biological origin.

B7.15 Carcinogens in spices, herbs, soups

Dried herbs and spices are often contaminated with alarmingly high levels of pesticides. Paprika and curry powders, as well as dried parsley, are particularly heavily contaminated, according to Greenpeace. "With a pinch of paprika or curry, as it lands on the currywurst, you sprinkle a toxic cocktail of up to 20 different chemicals, some of them carcinogenic, on your food," says Manfred Santen, a chemical expert at Greenpeace. Some currywursts contain hazardous substances such as the banned pesticide DDT (dichlorodiphenyltrichloroethane), chlorpyrifosethyl (a nerve toxin that inhibits cholinesterase) and carbendazim (which impairs reproduction).

Studies show that many spices, especially peppers, chili and curry spices are also contaminated with aflatoxins.

B7.16 Carcinogens in butter, margarine, oil

An excerpt from a report in the newspaper DIE ZEIT of June 17, 1954, shows us how industry at that time was most likely to blame for many people getting cancer by using a highly toxic chemical:

> "No field of medicine has been plowed through as deeply and thoroughly for decades as that of cancer research, but it has not yet succeeded in discovering the panacea. Modern science, however, has largely dissected [surrounded] this mortal enemy and has reached conclusions that leave room for hope. The cancer researcher Prof. Bauer-Heidelberg, one of the leading minds on this front, speaks of "cancer impulses foreign to the body", the causes of which lie in "our mechanized, chemized, denatured, modern world". Now here the views of the cancer researchers coincide with those of the nutritional physiologists, and only an ostrich brain could ignore this charge.
>
> It is directed primarily against the use of chemical substances that are harmful to health, such as those commonly used in the preservation, coloring, bleaching and conservation of our food and luxury foods. Some of these dyes from the group of hydrocarbons, the aniline derivatives, have even been described by research as clearly "cancerogenic"! In animal experiments, it has been determined that malignant tumors

> can almost certainly be produced by benzopyrene and cholanthrene under certain conditions. **An azo dye, dimethylaminoazobenzene,** was at the top of the list: it caused cancer in rats. And of all things, this azo dye was in circulation under the homely name of "butter yellow"; with it, in complete ignorance of its danger, our butter and margarine were dyed a beautiful, enticing golden yellow... The bombshell burst at the 55th conference of the German Society for Internal Medicine, which took place in Wiesbaden in May 1949. It was none other than Nobel Prize winner Prof. Butenandt, the director of the Max Plank Institute for Biochemistry. He revealed this hitherto fearfully guarded death secret of the "butter yellow". The excitement was tremendous, and people rightly asked: Are we being systematically poisoned? Are we all defenselessly at the mercy of the devious attacks of a poisonous corporation? Do federal and state authorities stand idly by and watch the cynical and public health-threatening violation of the provisions solemnly invoked in the Basic Law, which also apply to food monitoring? ...“
> (source: http://www.zeit.de/1954/24/werden-wir-vergiftet)

Hydrogenated oils

They are normally used to preserve industrially processed foods. But hydrogenated oils change the structure and flexibility of cell membranes throughout the body, and this can lead to several serious diseases, including cancer.

Time and again, experts warn against oil containing components of so-called polycyclic aromatic hydrocarbons (PAHs), carcinogenic substances. Some olive oils and foods preserved in oil, such as mussels, can also frequently contain such substances.

In addition to pesticide residues, an increased concentration of estrogens can also be found in butter. They originate from milk. It is known that cow's milk from factory farming contains hormones. This milk contains too much estrone sulfate. This estrogen compound is suspected of being able to cause testicular, prostate and breast cancer.

The substance group of glycidyl fatty acid esters is found in oils and fats. They contain a hazardous substance called glycidol. Glycidol is found in oil and margarine and is formed during the refining of fats. The chemical is used as a basic ingredient in the production of pharmaceuticals, sweeteners, flavors and insect poisons. However, the BfR (Federal Institute for Risk Assessment) and other specialist institutions unanimously classify the substance as carcinogenic. Hydrogenated fat is found in many products, such as deep-frying dough, convenience foods and ice cream. Infants in particular are at great risk, because the vegetable fat is also found in bottle feed.

Depending on which lobby study you are reading, margarine can be a good fat or a dangerous fat, even if it comes from vegetable oil (unsaturated fat) nowadays. However, the hardening of vegetable oils creates the dreaded saturated fatty acids. The fat-hardening process commonly used in margarine production leaves traces of toxic metals such as nickel or aluminum in the final product. Hardening vegetable oils can produce the so-called trans fatty acids, which have been shown to increase the risk of heart attacks and may be carcinogenic, even though nowadays the firm consistency of margarine is achieved by the process of "transesterification." Half-fat margarine must also be artificially preserved, which makes it even more unhealthy.

B7.17 Carcinogens in beverages: beer, wine, water, spirits, juices, lemonade, coke

- **Lemonades and coke**

Soft drinks or Coca-Cola contain many substances that can cause cancer. A study shows that soft drinks increase the risk of cancer by 87%. People who regularly drink sugary soft drinks (coke, soda and sweetened tea lemonade/iced tea) are more likely to develop pancreatic cancer! This was the finding of a study that followed more than 60,000 men and women over a 14-year period and was published in 2012.

Coca-Cola contains 4-methylimidazole, a carcinogenic coloring agent. A report titled "Cancer causing chemicals found in Coca-Cola coloring ingredient" at www.naturalnews.com/031383_caramel_coloring_cola.html states:

"The 'caramel coloring' used to color all the top cola brands isn't natural caramel coloring at all. Instead, it's made by reacting sugars with ammonia and sulfites at high temperatures. This reaction results in the formation of 2-methylimidazole and 4-methylimidazole, both of which are chemicals documented by the U.S. government to cause cancer in mammals."

Many soft drinks, including coke, fanta, lemonade, non-100% multivitamin juice, FUN ONE sugar-free, fitness cherry, iced tea, white tea & pear, green tea & grape, peach or rooibos tea, even juices, which are not 100% natural and at best directly pressed, are full of carcinogenic substances. Grape, peach or rooibos tea, also juices that are not 100% natural and best directly pressed are brimming with carcinogenic substances in all variations (dyes, sweeteners, preservatives, chemicals, such as 4-methylimidazole) and especially sugar.

The great danger often lies not in the individual substances, but in those that the manufacturers do not even tell the consumer about, which result from chemical reactions when different substances mix. The consumer is always told that ascorbic acid or sodium benzoate alone are not dangerous. But as is so often the case, the danger lurks in the combination of substances.

Toxic carcinogenic benzene in soft drinks

A shocking investigation of a soft drink test by the NDR magazine "Market" showed that many soft drinks contain benzene in dangerous amounts. Benzene is carcinogenic. The limit value was up to 6 times higher than that permitted amount for water. If the following substances are listed among the ingredients: Benzoic acid, (for example sodium benzoate, as a preservative) and ascorbic acid (vitamin C), this can cause benzene to form.

The substances styrene and acetophenone, which are hazardous to health and can cause cancer, were also discovered in the fashion drink bubble tea.

Drinks in plastic bottles are also a health hazard, as the plastic contains plasticizers that could be mixed into the drink. Plasticizers are known for their carcinogenic effect.

Diet drinks are dangerous sources of cancer. From one aspartame diet soda per day, the risk of cancer increases, more on this in Part B Chapter 7.21. "Diet foods, light products and dietary supplements".

- **Alcohol**

There is heated debate - even among researchers - about whether wine is harmful or perhaps even beneficial to health. But everyone is convinced that alcohol in general is cancer-promoting. Alcohol deprives the body of vitamins and magnesium, making it harder for the body to fight off free radicals. Free radicals are aggressive little electron particles. They are highly reactive molecules that react aggressively with other molecules. They cause body cells to age faster and are carcinogenic. Cancer, cardiovascular diseases, damage to the lens and retina of the eye and, to some extent, degenerative nerve diseases such as Alzheimer's and Parkinson's are now known as free radical diseases.

Heavy and regular alcohol consumption can promote cancer especially in the upper digestive tract (oral cavity, also pharynx, larynx and esophagus), colon, liver. Some studies say that alcohol can also play a role in breast cancer. A study from France was able to prove that a daily consumption of more than 80 grams of pure alcohol, about 2.5l of beer, increases the probability of developing esophageal cancer by 18 times. Together with cigarettes, the probability increases 44-fold. Apparently, the type of alcohol is not important for the development of cancer, but only the amount of alcohol drunk.

Many alcoholic beverages (liqueur wine, port, sherry and some fruit and grape brandies, wine, beer, etc.) contain the carcinogenic substance acetaldehyde. According to *Spiegel online,* the International Agency for Research on Cancer (IARC) rates acetaldehyde as clearly carcinogenic in animal experiments and as a probable elicitor of tumors in humans. Acetaldehyde can also be found in the food chain as a flavoring additive. The toxic decomposition product acetaldehyde has a damaging effect on human DNA, so it promotes the development of cancer.

Chemistry also plays a major role in the production of wine, as can be read in the book "Chemistry in Food". Pesticide residues (from grapes) are found in many wines. Some French wines were once contaminated by pesticide residues at concentrations up to a thousand times higher than the legal limits for tap water. This is extremely high and cannot pass through the body without harm. Sulfites are added to many wines, a preservative which can cause massive headaches or migraines. Sulfites are now also subject to mandatory labeling.

Dangerous plasticizers have even been found in wines...

- **Mineral water**

Many flavored waters do not contain real fruit. Water with crisp apple, tangy lemon or sweet strawberry that we see on the labels contain artificial flavors and lots of sugar. In a study, Stiftung Warentest (German consumer organization) discovered carcinogenic benzene in flavored mineral water.

What can also contaminate the mineral water are the plastic bottles. Chemicals such as plasticizers can leach out of them and contaminate the water without the consumer seeing it. During the production of PET bottles or during their storage, acetaldehyde can be formed as a degradation product and pass into the bottle contents. This substance is found particularly in carbonated beverages. The most expensive mineral water even performed worst in the test, according to a study by the Austrian consumer magazine *Konsument*.

B7. 18 Carcinogens in sugar, sweeteners, candy, chocolate, honey

Sugar can act like a poison. But the poison tastes so good and makes us happy with chocolates, sweets, ice cream, cake, yogurt, snacking, convenience foods, medications, drinks, etc. Every day it ends up in adults and children, even in babies, and yet it is one of the biggest killers of all, as studies from the USA show. Up to 35 million people die each year indirectly from sugar consumption.

Cancer loves sugar and especially industrial sugar (refined sugar). Industrial sugar is hidden in almost all ready meals, soft drinks, baked goods, baby and toddler food, often under different names such as sucrose, syrup, fructose, glucose, lactose, maltose E-number or even just a chemical formula. Many products are advertised as "no added sugar" but contain fructose as an ingredient. This is a clear lie, as fructose is sugar derived from corn. U.S. researcher Robert Lustig, who with his team conducted a study on the "toxic truth" of sugar (published in *Nature* Vol. 482 2012) said, "There is growing scientific evidence that fructose can cause quite a few chronic diseases and is toxic to the liver. [...] A little sugar may not be a problem, but a lot of sugar kills - albeit slowly."

Sugar makes you fat and cancer loves it where there is fat .

It has been scientifically proven that tumor cells need a lot of sugar to proliferate. Many researchers, such as Professor Lewis Cantley, of Harvard Medical School, suspect that in some cases, high sugar consumption causes cancer to develop in the first place. And refined sugar (industrially produced sugar) drives insulin levels up even faster and also causes cancer cells grow much faster than normal sugar.

Thanks to fructose, cancer cells can reproduce at lightning speed and spread throughout the human body, as scientists at the University of California, Los Angeles have proven in a study. Cheap syrup in drinks and convenience products consists of up to 90 percent fructose (corn syrup is preferred because it saves the industry a lot of money).

Sweeteners can be carcinogenic

Aspartame was on the CIA's list of biochemical warfare agents until the mid-1970s.

Many sweeteners, such as aspartame E951, cyclamate E952, (banned in the U.S. since 1969), saccharin E954, neotame E 961 and corn syrup (HFCS) are carcinogens. They are very popular with the industry because they are much cheaper than cane sugar and are found in thousands of products - from soft drinks to chewing gum and baked goods to medicines.

Since aspartame rightly came into disrepute (carcinogenic), the industry developed neotame. But neotame is merely a much better, or a much worse aspartame. In the European Union, neotame was approved on Jan. 12, 2010, as a sweetener and flavor enhancer, with the E number 961, for food. Since it is cheaper than aspartame, it is increasingly used by the industry. It is synthesized from aspartame and 3,3-dimethylbutyraldehyde is and 7,000-13,000 times sweeter than sugar and 30-60 times sweeter than aspartame (E951). Some studies show that neotame is much more toxic than aspartame.

The case of aspartame: Although the substance had already been approved as a sweetener for some time, studies on pregnant women and animal experiments raised suspicions that it could increase the risk of cancer. The European Food Safety Authority (EFSA) therefore re-evaluated aspartame. The EFSA experts did not find any evidence of a cancer-increasing effect. In a new review in 2013, the experts concluded that aspartame is safe as it is currently used in the EU, but as mentioned, many more independent studies show the opposite. As long as the industry funds many studies and many people groups and organizations, it will be very difficult to find the truth. Therefore, the only truth is simply CAUTION.

Refined sugars and sweeteners find their use especially in cookies, cake, lemonade, juices, chocolate, sauces, cereals, dipping sauces, baked goods, canned foods, dairy products and in many other popular, mostly industrially processed foods. Thus, they contribute powerfully and quietly quite unnoticed and with full enjoyment to people getting cancer.

- **Plastic particles in sweets**

We also find plasticizers in many sweets, in Nutella, butter, cheese and also whipped cream. An estimated 40% of our food contains toxic plasticizers. This was the conclusion reached by the NDR household program "Der große Küchen-Check".

The big shock came in 2010 when the German Federal Environment Agency identified the dangerous plasticizer DEHP, a phthalate, in Nutella. DEHP is one of the most dangerous plasticizers of all. Even then, the Federal Environment Agency tested 600 children for the plasticizer. The result: every child was contaminated with DEHP. The levels of some children were classified as extremely alarming by toxicologists who were consulted. In addition to suspected carcinogenic effects, studies have shown that plasticizers can attack the sex organs of men and make them infertile.

- **Honey**

Plant toxins in honey
Toxic alkaloids of the ragwort are said to be present in honey, according to Ökotest 2012. Honey is often contaminated with this cancer-causing plant substance. Raw honey from South and Central America is particularly affected, but small amounts of the toxin have also been found in European honey.

Ragwort is a yellow flowering weed that forms highly toxic alkaloids called pyrrolizidine alkaloids (PA). Large amounts can cause fatal illness (liver dysfunction). In animals, small amounts have been found to cause genetic damage and cancer. The Federal Institute for Risk Assessment (BfR) classifies this risk as serious if very large amounts of honey are consumed, and children may be at risk. Limit values do not yet exist for foodstuffs, but they do for medicines. One wonders how something can be strictly regulated (because dangerous) in medicines and arbitrarily present in food? The very fact that there is a limit for this substance in medicines is an indication of how dangerous it can be. PAs enter honey from the nectar of the plant via the bee. In high doses, this substance has a toxic effect and can cause severe liver damage.

- **Chocolate**

According to studies by the German Federal Institute for Risk Assessment (BfR), dark chocolate from South America in particular contains the substance cadmium. Cadmium is a heavy metal that damages the kidneys and bones and is highly carcinogenic. The higher the cocoa content, the higher the cadmium contamination.

B7.19 Carcinogens in teas, baby teas and Coffee: Is coffee more carcinogenic than a pesticide?

a. Tea

Issue 11/2014 of Stiftung Warentest reported on a study with 27 black teas: 19 Darjeelings and 8 Ceylon-Assam blends. Excessively high levels of potentially mutagenic and carcinogenic substances were found:

Pyrrolizidine alkaloids (PA)

Large amounts of this poison were found in Ceylon Assam tea from Kaufland, a German supermarket chain. Only one bag of this tea contained 0.9 micrograms! People of normal weight should not consume more than 0.4 micrograms of the substance per day. And with only one teabag, one already consumes twice as much.

There are no legal limits for PA in food in Germany, but surprisingly there is a legal limit in the pharmaceutical sector.

PAHs (polycyclic aromatic hydrocarbons)

Of the 27 teas tested, 12 had elevated levels of PAHs. PAHs are carcinogenic. Scientists claim that small amounts are not dangerous, but the amount makes the poison. And PAHs are unfortunately also found in many other products, such as smoked foods and the exhaust fumes we breathe in. Thus, we consume too many PAHs per day.

Other toxins found were: **Anthraquinone** (in 18 of the 19 Darjeelings). The poison enhances the dark coloration of the tea. The problem is that this substance causes cancer in animals, and it also has a very strong laxative effect. The recommended maximum level is 20 micrograms per kilogram of tea. In the tests, however, values up to 76 micrograms were found!

Mineral oil constituents (MOAH) were also detected in 15 teas. They are potentially carcinogenic

b. Carcinogenic substances in herbal and organic baby teas

The Federal Institute for Risk Assessment already warned in 2013 against excessive consumption of teas, because many of them contain carcinogenic substances! The office warned children, pregnant women and nursing mothers not to drink many herbal teas. It said: adults who drink more than five cups of herbal tea a day greatly increase the risk of cancer, studies show. Pyrrolizidine alkaloids are present in high amounts in tea, herbal tea and dried medicinal plants. For children, pregnant women and nursing mothers, the harmful substances in herbal tea could be dangerous. Scientists are finding "unexpectedly high levels of pyrrolizidine alkaloids," or PAs, in herbal and other teas.

The Federal Institute for Risk Assessment warned in summer 2013 that many herbal teas are contaminated with carcinogenic substances! The children, pregnant women and nursing mothers especially should not drink too much herbal tea. Adults who drink more than five cups of tea a day could do themselves a lot of harm.

In a study, the experts examined a total of 221 different commercially available herbal tea and tea samples as well as tea drugs (dried medicinal plants). These included baby fennel tea, chamomile tea, nettle tea, lemon balm tea and peppermint tea. High levels of the secondary plant compounds, pyrrolizidine alkaloids (PAs), were found in many of them, explained Andreas Hensel, president of the German Federal Office for Risk Assessment (BfR). Secondary plant compounds are substances that certain plants produce naturally as a defense against predators and microbial attack, and also act as growth regulators. Studies have shown that these substances cause cancer in animal experiments.

In an updated ÖKO-TEST (a few months later), 15 teas were examined, two conventionally produced and even three organic teas contained pyrrolizidine alkaloids. Pregnant women, nursing mothers and children should therefore not drink only tea, or consume it alternately with other beverages.

c. Coffee

Acrylamide

In 2014, the European Food Safety Authority published a report warning against acrylamide in roasted coffee. According to the German Federal Office of Consumer Protection and Food Safety (BVL), instant coffee contains up to almost 5000 micrograms of acrylamide per kilogram. Normal instant coffee contains up to 574 micrograms of acrylamide per kilogram, according to the BVL. With 3-4 cups of coffee a day, you can imagine the danger we are putting ourselves and our bodies in. Acrylamide is formed when food is prepared at temperatures of at least 150 degrees celsius.

Cancer caused by furan in coffee from fully automated coffee machines?

In 2006, an investigation by *Öko-Test magazine* found the carcinogenic substance acrylamide in all the coffees analyzed. Nine out of 18 roasted coffees contained more than the limit set by the testers. In addition, the mold toxin ochratoxin A and the pollutant furan were found.

Along with several other foods, coffee also contains the substance furan, which is suspected of causing cancer. Furan serves as a flavor carrier. In animal experiments, the substance, which is considered carcinogenic, was deposited in the liver of the animals. The ZDF (German public-service television broadcaster) documentary "Alles Bohne - Wie gut ist unser Kaffee?" reported on this. Furan gets into the coffee through the brewing method. According to the report, coffee brewed with a closed machine has higher furan levels than, for example, conventionally filtered coffee. Coffee from single-serving capsules is unhealthier than that from a filter machine. Furan is a substance that volatilizes easily. In filter coffee, it can do the same. In the capsule brewing method, it is trapped and remains in the coffee. Furan is formed when food is heated and therefore also in filter coffee. However, the concentration of this substance in capsules is much higher: 244 ng/ml compared to filter coffee with only 78 ng/ml.

In a German documentary it was reported how toxic the coffee plantations really are. It is not the coffee itself that is toxic, but the chemicals used. It can be assumed that the poisons used would also be detectable in the roasted coffee beans. One cannot really believe that all these poisons are actually completely broken down during roasting, when at the same time similar poisons are also detected in other products after processing.

Is a single cup of coffee more carcinogenic than a pesticide?

Some experts even believe that coffee is more dangerous than pesticides. This opinion is expressed by the well-known U.S. biochemist Bruce Ames in "Dietary Pesticides (99.99% all natural: carcinogens/mutagens/clastogens/coffee)". He opines that caffeic acid has been shown to be carcinogenic when fed in large quantities to rats and mice. One cup of coffee contains 10 milligrams of caffeic acid. He compares this amount to pesticide residue levels of some carcinogenic pesticides in food, which is less than 10 milligrams over the year. Bruce Ames was a researcher at the Children's Hospital of Oakland Research Institute (CHORI) and was director of the National Institute of Environmental Health Science at the University of California, Berkeley. He researched the link between folic acid deficiency and damage to DNA and chromosomes, which can lead to cancer and other diseases. In the 1970s, Ames invented the Ames test named after him and received more than 25 awards. I could not find any clear confirmation or refutation for his thesis on coffee in my research. But I have asked many researchers and research institutes and am still waiting for answers.

B7.20 Carcinogenic substances in convenience foods and frozen foods - cancer cocktail in industrial food

Conveniencefoods and frozen meals are dangerous sources of carcinogenic substances for the body.

Some of this food is made almost entirely from artificial products. For example, some use imitation food (pizza with cheese without milk, salami without meat). Ready meals contain too many dangerous preservatives, dyes, flavors, bad and too much fat, and artificially produced sugar, making them a real cancer cocktail for the body. All the poisons I have covered so far and many more that we don't even recognize and can't track are in convenience foods.

In 2012, there was a product recall at German supermarket chain Rewe: The retail group recalled a certain variety of frozen trout. Malachite green had been detected during an examination. According to the German Federal Institute for Risk Assessment (BfR), malachite green is a dye that is suspected of causing cancer and damaging genetic material. Another supermarket chain, PENNY, also recalled a variety of organic frozen broccoli because it contained the dangerous chemical chlorate. Chlorate is carcinogenic. While the products were recalled, how many people had eaten the fish or broccoli by then? The question is also which dangerous products are not detected at all, or if they are reported at all?

In 2013, an investigation by the Bavarian State Office for Health and Food Safety found pesticide residues in frozen soft fruit (strawberries, blueberries and raspberries).

One could cite so many examples that prove you have to be extra careful with frozen food.

The very dangerous plasticizer DEHP was also found in ready meals and canned foods as well as in fat-containing seasoning sauces. According to the study, mayonnaise or jarred vegetables and fish are also more heavily contaminated.

Frequent consumption of deep-fried frozen meals may increase the risk of prostate cancer. Studies show that people who eat a steady diet of convenience foods and frozen foods are more likely to develop cancer. A study from the U.S. showed that men who eat deep-fried frozen foods such as French fries, chicken nuggets or pastries baked in fat, such as donuts, at least once a week are 35 percent more at risk of prostate cancer than others who turn to these products at most once a month. Heating food at very high temperatures, as is the case with deep-frying, can produce acrylamide. This substance is suspected of causing cancer.

B7.21 Diet food, light products and dietary supplements

Almost all scientific studies warn against diet foods and diet drinks and light products. Diet drinks, like Diet Coke, are worse for your health than regular sugar-sweetened sodas. "Diet" soda and other diet drinks and foods may be carcinogenic.

All of these drinks, which are healthier at first glance, contain aspartame. Aspartame is a synthetically produced sweetener. As a food additive, it is declared as E 951. The substance is suspected of being highly carcinogenic. Aspartame is a widely used ingredient in many products such as soft drinks, confectionery, baked goods and dairy products.

From one aspartame diet soda per day, the risk of cancer increases!

The results of a recent aspartame study (a total of 77,218 women and 47,810 men participated in the studies, which ran over a period of 22 years) show: Already a can of diet soda (Cola light, iced tea without sugar, *sugarfree*, diet fruit spritzer or other light drinks) of 355 ml a day

- increases the risk of leukemia (blood cancer) by 42%.

- increases the risk of developing multiple myeloma (bone marrow cancer) by 102% in men
- increases the risk of non-Hodgkin's lymphoma (cancer of the lymph glands) in men by 31

In each case, compared with control subjects who did not drink diet sodas.

Already in the past, independent scientists found that the consumption of aspartame can lead to various diseases, such as cancerous tumors, lymphoma, leukemia, nerve damage, kidney failure, seizures and premature death.

Other substances, such as sucralose, supposedly derived from sugar, cause brain and nervous system dysfunction, migraines, cancer and weaken the immune system.

The consumption of saccharin is also not recommended.

Many diet foods contain additives that help build fat in the body. It has been proven that fat promotes cancer. Even though aspartame, saccharin and the like don't provide calories, they still cause you to get fat. Since the body naturally holds on to its calorie account, it demands a second and a third after one light yogurt. And inevitably, you get fat.

The funny thing is that many products call themselves "diet" because they contain sweeteners instead of normal sugar and are therefore low in calories, but in no way lead to weight loss.

The North-Rhine Westphalian Consumer Center has found carcinogenic substances such as sibutramine or the probably carcinogenic phenolphthalein in many diet products and light products, although they were declared as purely herbal.

B7.22 Genetically modified food

Many studies show that genetically modified foods can accelerate the growth of cancer cells. Possible effects of genetically modified products on health are far from professionally researched. Genetically modified crops are often heavily contaminated with pesticides. Substances and residues of genetically modified organisms have already been detected in the blood in several studies in animal experiments and in humans. A study from Canada confirmed that toxins from genetically modified organisms (GMOs) enter the human bloodstream. In 2011, this study by Aziz Aris and Samuel Leblanc was published in the Canadian journal *Reproductive Toxicology* "Maternal and fetal exposure to pesticides associated to genetically modified foods in Eastern township of Quebec, Canada" (in *Reproductive Toxicology*, 2011 May;31(4):528-33. Epub 2011 Feb 18). The study targeted maternal and fetal exposure to pesticides associated with genetically modified foods. The blood of 30 pregnant women and their babies and 39 nonpregnant women was analyzed for traces of glyphosate, glufosinate, and their major metabolites AMPA and 3-MPPA1, respectively, as well as for traces of Cry1Ab Toxinaus Bacillus thuringiensis. The women all resided in Sherbrooke, an urban region of Eastern Township in southern Quebec province. None of the test subjects had a partner who worked professionally with pesticides. This means that if anything was found, it had to have been forcibly ingested through the genetically modified foods such as soybeans and corn. In Canada, genetically modified foods are permitted.

From this study, one could be shocked to learn that some toxins that are carcinogenic and used to kill pests in genetic plants reach the bloodstream of women and unborn children almost 100%. Bttoxin has been found in the blood of 93% of pregnant women and 80% of unborn children. Many studies also show that a large number of the toxins in the gene products are not broken down by the body, as some studies claim. These toxins were found in the blood of animals that had previously consumed gene products such as corn, and in the blood of humans, as demonstrated by researchers in Canada.

Genetically modified products that are talked about a lot are soy, corn and rapeseed.

Is soy dangerous? Most soy plants are genetically modified. Some scientists at the University of Karlsruhe led by Professor Dr. Manfred Metzler, head of the Institute of Food Chemistry and Toxicology, have found that breakdown products of soy could cause cancer. Some breakdown products of soy resemble carcinogenic substances. They are said to be plant hormones called "phytoestrogens." The scientist: "This means that these substances and some of their breakdown products are potentially carcinogenic." However, these are not yet conclusive results.

Genetically modified foods such as genetically modified corn are contaminated with both herbicidal active ingredients such as glyphosate and toxins such as the Bt-protein (this toxin is supposed to protect the plant from predators from the inside out; it acts like a pesticide. The plants themselves thus produce toxin). How dangerous such substances are has already been proven in laboratory rats. In 2012, a genetically modified corn study from Caen, France, showed that lab rats fed genetically modified corn for their entire lives developed tumors and also suffered from organ damage. They died earlier than the other rats. The human body does not seem to be able to break down such toxins.

Glufosinate, in particular, is considered a risk factor for human reproductive function. An opinion from the European Food Safety Authority (EFSA) classifies glufosinate, a precursor of 3-MMPA, as carcinogenic. In Japan, studies showed that glufosinate provoked premature births in rats.

As I can see from my research and responses to my inquiries, definitive studies that incriminate or absolve (GMOs) have not been completed. However, as mentioned above, there are some indications to consider certain substances used in NGOs as dangerous. As in other areas where a lot of money is implemented, studies will confirm one way or the other depending on the interest.

B7.23 Chemicals and poison in organic farming

Generally, it is said that organic products (meat, vegetables, fruit and co) must be produced without genetic modification, chemical fertilizers and pesticides. Unfortunately, this is not always the case.

Organic is not always organic. Not all organic products are the same. Especially the organic brands of the supermarkets can contain carcinogenic substances. Dioxin has already been found in organic eggs!

Many organic products are sprayed with pesticides just like conventional products.

One danger with organic products is mold. To combat this, conventional poisons are sprayed, which unfortunately can be found in some organic products at the end consumer.

Dangerous additives are also used in many organic products; it is therefore very important to read the ingredients on the packaging carefully. Some have been proven to be carcinogenic, and here the consumer needs to know that organic products may also contain up to seven additives without labeling. This means that there can be the same additives in organic products as in conventional products, but they can still be called "organic." For example:

- Carrageenan: found in organic dairy products. Carrageenan is extracted from red algae and is extremely controversial, as the substance has led to ulcers and changes in the immune system in animal tests
- Nitrite curing salt: certain organic sausages contain nitrite curing salt, which can form carcinogenic nitrosamines.
- Ascorbic acid (vitamin C)

In Germany, organic associations such as "Demeter" do not use such dangerous additives.

In the past, carcinogenic substances have repeatedly been found in organic products. The consumer organization Foodwatch warned about acrylamide in some organic potato chips: Acrylamide is carcinogenic.

Another case occurred in 2007, when Stiftung Warentest found a particularly high concentration of the carcinogenic substance benzopyrene in "Bio Negro" dark chocolate. Benzopyrene belongs to the carcinogenic group of substances known as polycyclic aromatic hydrocarbons (PAHs). The product was withdrawn from the market at that time.

In 2013, Stiftung Warentest found the potentially carcinogenic substance anthraquinone in Pura Pesto from Basilico Genovese D.O.P. with a best-before date of July 4, 2014.

B7.24 Carcinogenic substances through food packaging: Plastic in our food

Many packaging materials contain substances that are ingested by people through food and lead to serious health conditions such as cancer.

"Besides pesticide residues from agricultural production, plastic packaging and containers are a second major source of endocrine-disrupting chemicals in our food." So says a brochure from Global 2000, the Austrian environmental organization. Plastic products made of polycarbonate (PC), polyvinyl chloride (PVC) should be avoided.

Endocrine disruptors and plasticizers

Among the most common endocrine-disrupting chemicals found in plastics that are carcinogens are phthalates. They are found as plasticizers in polyvinyl chloride (PVC) and bisphenol A (BPA), the starting material for polycarbonate and epoxy resins. BPA can also be found in plastics such as polyamide, silicone and latex. It is almost impossible to live without coming into contact with these chemicals as they are almost everywhere: in cell phones, CDs, DVDs, toys, etc. But it is strongly recommended to avoid food packaging, cash register receipts and food cans made of these materials (PVC films, for example). The inside of food cans is lined with a thin plastic layer. This is almost always made of epoxy resins, which release BPA into the food. It can be done differently, as Japan shows with cans lined with PET instead of BPA. Phthalates and bisphenol A are detectable in human blood, urine, breast milk and the umbilical cord blood of newborns. Pacifiers made with BPA are dangerous to babies. Since BPA is also absorbed through the skin, infants should avoid contact with products containing BPA. When purchasing household foils, make sure they are phthalate-free (PVC free).

Dangerous plasticizer DEHP in foodstuffs

In addition to the cancer risk, plasticizers are also suspected of promoting diabetes and asthma. The toxic substances could even lead to respiratory diseases. Plasticizers can also make people infertile. A study by the Federal Environment Agency showed that 50% of all men aged 18 to 23 in Germany have only limited fertility. Nutella, butter, cheese and whipped cream, Géramont soft cheese (80 micrograms per kg), Bertolli pesto (240 µg per kg) and Kerrygold butter (520 µg per kg) and many others also contain toxic plasticizers. This was the conclusion reached by the NDR household program "Der große Küchen-Check".

The toxins get from the packaging into the food and later through the food into our bodies....

Mineral oil residues

Mineral oil components also get into food through the packaging. Printed newsprint is also used for the production of cardboard from recycled wastepaper. Most newsprint inks contain mineral oils. These are not 100% removed during processing and thus enter food packaging. Other possible routes for oils to enter bodies are lubricants from food production equipment. The BfR assumes that especially in the case of dry foods with a large surface area, such as flour, semolina, rice, breadcrumbs or breakfast cereals, a transfer of mineral oils from the packaging to the food is to be expected.

Aluminum

Aluminum can be found in food packaging. Scientists agree, aluminum is threatening to every form of life if it is ingested in larger quantities and over a longer period of time. Especially children should not drink too many juices. Aluminum also enters food through contact with packaging or containers. Storage tanks containing aluminum in particular release aluminum when they come into contact with the acidic fruit juices and fruit wines.

B7.25 Food imitations, new sources of cancer?

In addition to ham substitutes and artificial cheese, many other food imitations end up with consumers.

Many experts and consumer advocates consider the imitations to be harmful to health. In order for the product to taste somewhat like the original products, massive amounts of additives are used, thus increasing the concentration of carcinogenic pollutants and the risk of contracting cancer because of it, so it is assumed. There are no conclusive studies on this yet.

B8 What other diseases are promoted by poor nutrition?

A poor diet and an unhealthy lifestyle promote not only the development of cancer, but also many other diseases: from colds to diabetes, to migraines.

A healthy lifestyle and the right diet, on the other hand, can prevent diseases, cure them or support healing.

Part 2

How nutrition cures cancer:

CANCER

I want to defeat you

I can defeat you

I will defeat you!

That's why I'm starting now!

Foods and an African-inspired diet that will protect you from and fight cancer!

Introduction: Connection between nutrition, food and health – a small, personal story

My mother has not gone to the doctor for over 50 years because she is hardly ever sick; my brother and sister, who both studied in Germany and now live back in Cameroon, have not knocked on a doctor's door for decades, and their children have never been to the doctor either - they are not against medicine or doctors, but they all enjoy such robust health that they are hardly ever sick. Through their diet, they fight and prevent disease quite automatically.

From my childhood in Africa over 40 years ago, I learned that good nutrition and the right food choices are half the health. My parents used to tell us, "eat well and God will keep you healthy." There is a lot of truth in that phrase.

I grew up in a so-called "modern" family, but our diet remained African. It struck us even then that friendly families, at a similar social level, frequently complained of health problems; we were amazed at how often parents and children fell ill and had to go to the doctor. A neighbor asked us why we were so rarely sick, his children had to take medication all the time, three of the five children needed glasses at an early age, the two oldest had bronchitis all the time and all were overweight. My father suspected that the ailments were related to the Western style of eating that the family had adopted. It was generally seen as a sign of social success to try to live like Europeans and to distance oneself from the healthy African diet. I remember that many people made fun of us and criticized my parents because it was not appropriate for our social standing to always eat so African - one should show that one had "arrived"!

In the family in question, the warm African breakfast was not served anymore, but white bread with cheese, super-sweetened canned milk from Nestlé, cocoa powder in which there is almost no real cocoa, canned fish, and so on. At lunchtime and in the evening, there was only rice, dishes breaded with white flour, canned ready meals, French fries with mayonnaise and ketchup, various yogurts and puddings as dessert, water as a drink had disappeared and was replaced by coke and fanta - all purchased in the supermarkets of the "whites".

Yes, that was the diet of the successful people in Cameroon. They thought that this made them "civilized", just like the Europeans. My father advised the neighbor to do without all these foods for at least 3 months and to return to the original, African diet, with lots of fresh vegetables and fruit, with spices, ginger, hardly any white flour and even less sugar and the total renunciation of canned milk. Then he was to see how things turned out. Sure enough, after a few weeks, many of the family's ailments had disappeared on their own and the children hardly needed any medication. The change in diet - away from industrially produced food - had made the family healthy again.

During my research for my anti-aging book, I read a lot about people who lived or still live long and healthy. I talked to people who were still fit in old age without medical help. And I noticed a common denominator: they all ate a very healthy diet, especially with very little so-called "industrial food." They hardly drank any coke or soda, they ate little white flour and dairy products from conventional animal husbandry, fast food was practically forbidden among them, and they hardly drank any coffee. They ate the way I knew it from my childhood, and what was called "uncivilized and primitive".

The normal eating habits of my home country Cameroon are, strictly speaking, already a diet program and medical cure in one. The food is varied, rich in vitamins and minerals, alkaline, contains lots of fresh, pesticide-free vegetables and fruits, it is well and spicy seasoned, with chili, ginger and herbs, there is a lot of fish and healthy beef (the cattle in Cameroon only eat grass) and the food is prepared with lots of healthy vegetable oil - preferably palm, peanut or coconut oil. With such a diet, the food becomes natural remedies for body and soul and one is holistically healthy. Many diseases that people in Western countries suffer from are unknown in large parts of Africa, because from a very early age, care is taken to eat healthy food in order to prevent diseases.

What is crucial for the natural effectiveness of food against cancer?

After evaluating many studies and talking to patients, natural doctors and conventional doctors, I found that people whose diet was particularly varied and predominantly alkaline, with large amounts of spices and different, antioxidant foods, had a lower risk of cancer, or that if they did develop cancer, they had a better chance of recovery. This was the best way for them to support therapy.

Cooking without spices and herbs would already be a gross negligence against one's own health, because herbs and spices are and partly act like real medicines.

Decisive for the natural effectiveness of food is not only the quality of food, its origin and its preparation, but also the selection (which food) and most importantly an overall change in diet. That meant a single food or a single vitamin alone would hardly show any effect. Only the mixture of many different good foods and the interaction between them is the key to success, according to my research. This is how you can beat cancer.

C. Healthy diet - the basis of the fight against cancer

C1 Basic prerequisite for a type of nutrition that heals

The basic requirement for food to heal and help is to know certain things and apply that knowledge. It is important to have a basic attitude towards healthy food. Alkaline foods, healthy oils and foods rich in vitamins and minerals play the central role.

I enrich readers by including many exotic foods that are available for purchase here, but that many are not yet aware of and that have miraculous healing powers.

C2 Healthy intestinal flora: First prerequisite for healthy weight loss and successful disease prevention

All regeneration, detoxification and healing begins in the intestines, which means through nutrition. Just like losing weight. This insight has a central importance in African medicine.

To lose weight in a healthy way and burn fat, a healthy flora and intestinal mucosa is required. If the intestine is not in order, healing through food and sustainable weight loss is hardly possible, because in the intestine the breakdown, processing and absorption of nutrients takes place and from there they are then distributed throughout the body.

Herbs are the best way to cleanse your intestines and get healthy. In my home country, there is a sauce with over 20 spices that you can drink or eat with corn porridge. This sauce (nkui) really washes the stomach and eliminates intestinal mucosa inflammation.

Herbs fight pathogens in the intestine, intestinal infections, intestinal spasms, diarrhea, strengthen the immune defenses of the intestine and regenerate it, stimulate the formation of acid. These are, for example, oregano, basil, gentian, anise, celery, dill, nasturtium.

Probiotics can also be used to successfully achieve this result. Probiotic lactic acid bacteria are contained in sauerkraut, for example.

Other foods that cleanse the intestinal flora and let it regenerate are:

- Ginger
- Onion
- Garlic
- If one were to use these three foods more often in food preparation, preferably together, one would hardly need to do anything special. It would be enough. Besides:
- Chili peppers, especially fresh round pods. They are sometimes green, sometimes yellow or red. They contain an active ingredient called capsaicin. This protects the stomach much better than many drugs. In Africa, chili is used to treat the sick intestinal flora and this simply by cooking spicy or making the leaves of the plants into tea and drink.
- African carbohydrates, see chapter C 3.10.18
- Okra
- Bitter leaf and all bitter vegetables, such as chicory, artichokes and salsify.
- Very effective: tea from guava and mango leaves and bark, if you want.
- Certain fruits like apples (Braeburn), blueberries, blackberries, green mango, bananas - they have a disinfecting effect
- Vitamin C via sea buckthorn juice
- natural "antibiotics", such as cold-spun bee honey; relieve inflammation in the intestines
- Vegetable oils are very important in the restoration of healthy intestinal flora
- Teas like peppermint, chamomile, ginger

In my book "Healthy and healed with the food pharmacy" you can learn even more about it.

Fasting can also clean up your intestinal flora. In my own experience, regular fasting therapies usually work better than medication.

C3 What foods make us healthy and act like pills?

C3.1 Foods rich in vitamins: table of important vitamins with their functions and a list of foods in which they can be found

I have not included all the foods here so that the list still remains clear. Many of the foods can be easily found in the local market. There are exotic foods like moringa or okra that contain a lot of different vitamins. I will write a separate book about these tropical fruits and foods.

Vitamins are divided into two groups:

1 Fat-soluble vitamins: A, D, E, K

2 Water-soluble vitamins: B group and C

(*** With the help of Jumk.de)

Name	Main occurrence	Effectiveness	Deficiency
Vitamin A (retinol)	Cod liver oil, liver, kidney, milk products, butter, egg yolk, as pro vitamin A in carrots	Normal growth, function and protection of skin, eyes and mucous membrane	Growth arrest, night blindness

Name	Main occurrence	Effectiveness	Deficiency
Provitamin A Beta carotene	In yellow-orange and green fruit: carrot, apricot, spinach, melon, pumpkin parsley, kale, sweet potato	Precursor of vitamin A, antioxidants - make free radicals harmless - support the immune system	Accelerates aging process
Folic acid	Liver, egg yolk, apricots, beans, green leafy vegetables, carrots, avocados, melon, oranges, whole grain products	Essential for growth & cell division, especially for the formation of red blood cells. Especially important for women of fertile age. Promotes the development of the nervous system in the unborn child	Increased risk of cancer, fatigue, digestive problems, nervousness, poor memory, insomnia, confusion, miscarriages, shortness of breath

Name	**Main occurrence**	**Effectiveness**	**Deficiency**
Vitamin B1 (thiamine)	Wheat germ, whole grains, peas, heart, pork, yeast, oat flakes, liver, brown rice,	Important for the nervous system, poor performance, pregnancy, mosquito protection (high dosage), energy - production in the body, influences carbon hydrate metabolism, important for thyroid function	severe muscle and nerve disorders, fatigue, digestive disorders, dropsy, heart failure, cramps, paralysis, tingling in arms and legs
Vitamin B2 (riboflavin)	Dairy products, meat, whole grains, cheese, eggs, liver, sea fish, green leafy vegetables, whey powder	Important for body growth, utilization of fats, protein & carbohydrates, good for skin, nails & eyes, important energy provider, oxygen transport	(rare) skin inflammation, brittle fingernails, anemia, corneal opacity

Name	Main occurrence	Effectiveness	Deficiency
Vitamin B3 (**niacin**, nicotinic acid)	Barm, peanuts, peas, liver, poultry, fish, lean meat	Build-up and breakdown of fat, protein and carbohydrates, good sleep	Skin and mucous membrane inflammations, headaches, tremors, sleep disturbances, dizziness, depression, tingling and numbness in the limbs.
Vitamin B5 (**pantothen acid**)	Liver, vegetables, wheat germ, asparagus, meat, crab, sunflower seeds, pumpernickel	Against graying, hair loss, hair and mucous membrane diseases, is needed for the breakdown of fat, proteins and carbohydrates	Nerve dysfunction-, poor wound healing, early graying, weakened immune system
Vitamin B6 (pyridoxine)	Bananas, nuts, whole grains, yeast, liver, potatoes, green beans, cauliflower, carrots	Helps with motion sickness, nerve pain, liver damage, premenstrual syndrome, protein digestion, together with folic acid the	(rather rarely) intestinal problems, bad skin, fatigue, brittle corners of the mouth

Name	**Main occurrence**	**Effectiveness**	**Deficiency**
		most important - pregnancy hormone, detoxification	
Vitamin B7 (**biotin**, vitamin H)	Liver, meat, cauliflower, mushrooms, whole grain products, egg, avocado, spinach, milk	Skin diseases, hair growth damage, liver damage, supports metabolic processes, is needed together with vitamin K to build up blood clotting factors, supports carbohydrate and fatty acid metabolism for skin and mucous membranes	Fatigue, skin inflammation, muscle pain, hair loss, nausea, depression
Vitamin B9 (**folic acid** Vitamin M)	Liver, wheat germ, pumpkin, mushrooms, spinach, avocado	Liver damage, cell division, healing and growth of muscles and cells, protein metabolism, tissue formation	Anemia, digestive disorders, hair, bone and cartilage growth disorders

Name	Main occurrence	Effectiveness	Deficiency
Vitamin B12 (cobalamin)	Liver, milk, egg yolk, fish, meat, oysters, curd, barm	Structure of cell nucleus, formation of red blood cells, nerve pain, skin and mucous membrane diseases, liver damage	Anemia, nervous disorders, changes in the lungs and spinal cord
Vitamin C (ascorbic acid)	Rose hips, sea buckthorn, citrus, currant, potatoes, peppers, tomatoes, cabbage, spinach, vegetables, radish	Anti-inflammatory and anti-bleeding, promotes defense, protects cells from chemical destruction, activates enzymes, builds connective tissue, bone and tooth enamel, faster wound healing, stabilizes the psyche	Bleeding gums, fatigue, joint pain, headache, poor wound healing, lack of appetite, scurvy, poor performance

Name	**Main occurrence**	**Effectiveness**	**Deficiency**
Vitamin D (calciferol)	Cod liver oil, liver, milk, egg yolk, butter, sea fish, mushrooms, avocado, herring	Regulates calcium and phosphate balance, bone formation, promotes calcium absorption	Bone deformity and softening, osteomalacia, increased susceptibility to infections, muscle weakness
Vitamin E (tocopherol)	Sunflower, corn, soybean and wheat germ oil, nuts, flaxseed, black salsify, hot peppers, cabbage, avocado	Strengthens the immune system, anti-inflammatory, cell renewal, protection against radicals, regulates cholesterol levels and hormone balance, important for blood vessels, muscles and reproductive organs	(rare) visual impairment, fatigue, muscle wasting, unpleasure, reproductive difficulties

Name	Main occurrence	Effectiveness	Deficiency
Vitamin K (phyllo-quinone)	Cress, liver, kale, kiwi, green vegetables, onions, oatmeal, tomatoes, eggs	Required for the formation of blood clotting factors	High doses of vitamins A and E counteract vitamin K

C3.2 Mineral-rich foods: Table of important minerals and trace elements and which natural foods contain them

The human body cannot be healthy without minerals. Doctors attribute the cause of many diseases to a lack of minerals. However, the human body cannot produce natural minerals such as potassium or magnesium on its own but can only absorb them through food.

Many scientific studies show that our body cannot utilize artificial minerals, therefore the best and proper supply is only possible with natural minerals.

*** Thanks for the help of www.orthoknowledge.eu/vitamine-tabel/

Name	Main occurrence	Effectiveness	Deficiency

C3 What foods make us healthy and act like pills?

Name	Main occurrence	Effectiveness	Deficiency
Boron B	Pears, prunes, raisins, legumes, apples, tomatoes	Helps prevent calcium loss and demineralization of bones. May improve memory and cognitive functions	Bone diseases, growth problems, arthritis, fungal and bacterial infections
Calcium Ca	Dairy products, legumes, vegetables, tofu, salmon, nuts	Building block of bones and teeth. Required for nerve and muscle functions	Bone decalcification-, poor dentition and bone structure, allergies, high blood pressure, migraines, heart problems
Chloride Cl	Table salt, seaweed, fish products, seaweed, olives, seawater, water of the Great Salt Lake	Regulates the acid-base balance in the blood, forms a chemical -bond with sodium and potassium. Stimulates liver function. Plays an important role in digestion	Premature hair and tooth loss
Chromium Cr	Whole grain products, meat, fish, liver, barm, mushrooms, egg yolks	Acts in the body as a glucose tolerance factor (GTF) that stimulates insulin action	Irritability, depressiveness, hypoglycemia, high cholesterol, anxiety, diabetes

Name	Main occurrence	Effectiveness	Deficiency
Iron **Fe**	Seaweed, mussels, oysters, nuts, cocoa powder, red meat, egg yolks	Component of red blood cells. Important for oxygen transport - through the body and for the immune system. Is a component of various metabolic enzymes	Anemia, poor hearing, menstrual pain, restless legs syndrome, fatigue
Iodine **I**	Fish, crustaceans and shellfish, pineapple, seaweed, raisins, dairy products	Formation of hormones in the thyroid gland. To maintain the health of the skin, hair and nails	Thyroid problems, goiter, tough mucosa

Name	Main occurrence	Effectiveness	Deficiency
Potassium K	Nuts, green vegetables, avocados, bananas, soybean meal, potatoes, Great Salt Lake water	Forms, together with sodium and chloride, the vital electrolyte salts essential for fluid balance in the body. Involved in muscle function, nerve conduction, heart activity and energy production. Stabilizes the internal cell structure.	Vomiting, drowsiness, muscle weakness and paralysis, low blood pressure, drowsiness, confusion, extreme fatigue
Copper Cu	Avocados, offal, beet syrup, crustaceans, oysters, kidneys, egg yolks, fish, legumes	Component (with zinc and manganese) of the antioxidant enzyme system. Required for pigment synthesis and iron metabolism	Anemia, edema, bleeding, problems with skin pigmentation, hair problems, mild irritability, loss of sense of taste, loss of appetite

Name	Main occurrence	Effectiveness	Deficiency
Magnesium Mg	Water from the Great Salt Lake in Utah - one of the richest deposits of natural magnesium. Brown rice, soybeans, nuts, fish, legumes, whole grains, barm, green leafy vegetables, dark chocolate	Involved in over 200 functions in the body. Plays a role in bone formation, energy production and muscle and nerve functions. Also important for heart and blood circulation. Component of many enzymes. Co-factor for vitamins B and C	Irregular pulse, lack of drive, kidney stones, asthma, osteoporosis, depression and anxiety, PMS, period pain, fibromyalgia, glaucoma, diabetes, low endurance (especially in athletes), insomnia, migraines, gum problems, high cholesterol, high blood pressure, hearing loss, prostate problems
Manganese Mn	Whole grains, nuts, vegetables, liver, tea, carrots	Component (with zinc and copper) of the antioxidant enzyme system. Required for bone formation, joints and the nervous system	Dermatitis, poor memory function, epilepsy, anemia, diabetes, heart trouble, arthritis

Name	Main occurrence	Effectiveness	Deficiency
Molybdenum Mo	Buckwheat, wheat germ, legumes, liver, whole grains, eggs	Involved in the metabolism of sulfur-containing - amino acids and in the production of uric acid. Antioxidant. Required for the synthesis of taurine	Male impotence, mild irritability, irregular pulse
Sodium Na	Table salt, shellfish, carrots, artichokes, beets, dried beef	Ensures that the muscles and nerves function properly	Sunstroke, drowsiness due to heat
Phosphorus P	Meat, yeast, whole grain products, cheese, nuts, soy, fish	Required for the overall structure of the body. Component of ATP, the energy carrier in the muscles	Confusion, lack of appetite, weakness, irritability, speech problems, decreased resistance to infections, anemia

Name	Main occurrence	Effectiveness	Deficiency
Selenium Se	Tuna, herring, - tomatoes, onions, broccoli, wheat germ and bran	Acts as an antioxidant and provides protection against signs of aging. Contributes to the prevention of immune diseases	Decreased immunity and resistance to infections, decreased fertility in males, age spots, retarded growth
Vanadium V	Parsley, radishes, lettuce, bone meal, crabs	Significant for the electrolyte balance. Action potentials of muscles and nerves. Bones and teeth	Unknown
Zinc Zn	Meat, mushrooms, seeds, nuts, oysters, eggs, whole grains, barm	Guardian of the immune system. Indispensable for the structure and function of cell membranes. Required for reproduction and blood sugar levels	Male infertility, skin rash, arthritis, ulcers, growth problems, allergies, - alcohol dependency

C3.3 Antioxidant-rich foods fight the cause of chronic inflammation like cancer

Antioxidants are chemical compounds that specifically prevent the unwanted oxidation of other substances. They are radical scavengers. Free radicals attack cells and cause oxidative stress. This is considered to be partly responsible for aging and is associated with the development of a number of diseases.

Antioxidants protect the body from these attacks by interrupting the chain reactions of free radicals. They thus prevent oxidative stress and avert cell damage.

Antioxidants can do much more. They

- offer protection from environmental pollutants
- offer protection against Alzheimer's disease, lung diseases such as asthma or bronchitis, cancer, heart disease and strokes, arteriosclerosis and protect the eyes against macular degeneration (retinal damage leading to progressive vision loss)
- lower the cholesterol level
- slow down the aging process
- support the body in the fight against damage caused by cigarette smoke, alcohol, poor nutrition, stress,
- and much more

Antioxidants are found in many groups including:

Vitamins, minerals, trace elements, enzymes and secondary plant substances.

a. Occurrence of natural antioxidants

Occurrence of natural antioxidants	
Compound(s)	**Food with high content**
Vitamin C (ascorbic acid)	Fresh fruit and vegetables
Vitamin E (tocopherols, tocotrienols)	Vegetable oils
Polyphenolic antioxidants (resveratrol, flavonoids)	Tea, coffee, soy, fruit, olive oil, cocoa, cinnamon, oregano, red wine, pomegranate
Carotenoids (lycopene, beta-carotene, lutein)	Fruits, vegetables, eggs.

(Source: Wikipedia)

Breast milk is also a source of antioxidants for the baby. Several antioxidants are passed on to the infant as a component of breast milk to exert their effect.

b. Synthetic antioxidants

There are not only natural antioxidants, they are also produced synthetically. However, these can pose health risks. Cancer-promoting effects have already been proven in many studies. In animal studies, some antioxidants have been shown to impair growth and the body's defense against infections. Allergies can also occur in humans. It is therefore advisable to consume as few of these artificial radical scavengers as possible.

Synthetic antioxidants permitted in food:

Just because a ready meal says "antioxidant" on its packaging doesn't mean you should think you're doing something good

E 220 Sulfur dioxide	**E 322** Lecithin
E 221 Sodium sulfite	**E 330** Citric acid
E 222 Sodium hydrogen sulfite	**E 331 & E 332** Salts of citric acid
E 223 Sodium disulfide	**E 331** Sodium citrate
E 224 Potassium disulfide	**E 332** Potassium citrate
E 226 Calcium sulfite	**E 385** Calcium disodium EDTA
E 227 Calcium hydrogen sulfite	**E 450** Diphosphates
E 228 Potassium hydrogen sulfite	**E 450a** Disodium diphosphate
E 270 Lactic acid	**E 450b** Trisodium diphosphate
E 300 Ascorbic acid	**E 450c** Tetrasodium diphosphate
E 301 Sodium L-ascorbate	**E 450d** Dipotassium diphosphate
E 302 Calcium L-ascorbate	**E 450e** Tetrapotassium diphosphate
E 304 Ascorbic acid ester	**E 450f** Dicalcium diphosphate
E 306 Tocopherol	**E 450g** Calcium dihydrogen di-phosphate
E 307 Alpha tocopherol	**E 451** Triphosphates
E 308 Gamma tocopherol	**E 451a** Pentasodium triphosphate
E 309 Delta tocopherol	**E 451b** Pentapotassium triphosphate
E 310 Propyl gallate	**E 452** Polyphosphate
E 311 Octyl gallate	**E 452a** Sodium polyphosphate
E 312 Dodecyl gallate	**E 452b** Potassium polyphosphate
E 315 Erythorbic acid	**E 452c** Sodium calcium polyphosphate
E 316 Sodium erythorbate	**E 452d** Calcium polyphosphate
E 319 Tert-butylhydroquinone (TBHQ)	**E 512** Tin II chloride
E 320 Butylated hydroxyanisole	
E 321 Butylated hydroxytoluene	

for your health!

Note: Synthetic antioxidants are used in the following processed foods (only an excerpt):

- Infant formula
- Dairy products: cheese
- Greasy food, saturated fats (trans fats), high calorie food, convenience food, fast food, frozen food, bad oil, mayonnaise and salad dressing, animal fat, pizza, breaded food, etc.
- Meat and meat substitutes: Meat products, sausages, smoked meats, cured meats, offal, cutlets, roasted meats, meat loaf, tofu, but also fish and canned fish
- Dried or frozen fish with red skin, salted dried fish
- Nuts with shells
- Sweets, ice cream, jam, chewing gum
- Fruits and vegetables: peeled potatoes, frozen potato products, dried potato products, cut and packaged vegetables and fruits, dried tomatoes, white vegetables dried or frozen, dried fruits, canned fruits
- Sweetened beverages: fruit drinks, fruit nectar, sweetened juices or sodas such as coke and soda; tea and coffee with sugar, energy drinks
- Wheat: white flour, cake, egg pasta, bread, pasta, cake mixes, yeast
- Edible oils, edible fats

C3.4 Omega-3 fatty acids - important components of food: Which foods contain the polyunsaturated fatty acids?

Omega-3 fatty acids belong to the polyunsaturated fatty acids, such as DHA and are important and necessary components of our diet and they are especially needed in the brain. The human brain is largely composed of DHA, which is needed to strengthen brain performance and fight against numerous diseases, such as Alzheimer's disease, heart attacks, dementia, thrombosis and ADHs, it also helps against obesity.

Omega-3 fatty acids are further needed for: the production of hormones, the synthesis of protein, the fight against inflammation and infection, the formation of the body's own defense cells. They protect the heart, lower blood lipid levels, blood pressure, reduce blood sugar levels and much more.

DHA can be supplied both through the diet, especially through oils of fatty marine fish, such as mackerel, herring, eel and salmon, and synthesized in the human organism from the essential alpha-linolenic acid.

Good foods that contain omega-3 fatty acids:

- Fish: salmon, herring, tuna, mackerel, eel
- Oil: Hemp oil, linseed oil, walnut oil, algae oil, rapeseed oil, soybean oil, these do not contain DHA and EPA, but their precursor, the omega-3 fatty acid ALA (alpha-linolenic acid). The body can convert this precursor into DHA and EPA. 20 grams of rapeseed oil (about two tablespoons) correspond to about 1 to 1.5 grams of omega-3 fatty acids. This would be sufficient for the daily requirement.
- Flaxseed, walnuts

Prolonged intake of very high doses of omega-3 fatty acids from dietary supplements can lead to health problems, such as the increase of cholesterol levels, weakening of the immune system, increase of infectious diseases and inflammation-related diseases, nausea, vomiting, etc.

C3.5 Abundant vegetable oil is healthy and an effective anti-cancer agent

Oil does not automatically make you fat. Oil is a healing agent. Without oil, the body cannot function at all. What oil does in our body works on the same principle as oil in the engine of a car. Without oil, our body "rusts".

A good balance of saturated and unsaturated oils is very good for the body.

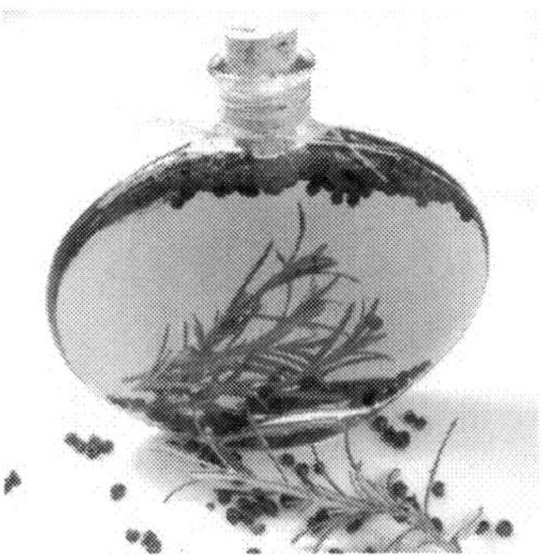

I am not okay with how some nutritionists want us to believe that oil is unhealthy. What primitive people use for thousands of years and with which they also fight diseases, cannot be unhealthy today. One should compare to see the truth for oneself. In the countries of Africa and Asia, for example in Cameroon or China, food is prepared in abundant vegetable oil. There is a lot of deep frying. But in these countries, we see people with the fewest civilization diseases associated with fat. And in Western countries, we find people who often suffer from such diseases, although they use very little oil from plants.

During my teaching in Africa, I learned that the body needs the combination of saturated and unsaturated vegetable oils and even animal fat from animal meat.
It just must be healthy oils and healthy animals.

I learned early on that every cell in our body (brain, bone, skin, muscle, etc.) relies on fatty acids.

As I have already explained, oil is not unhealthy just because it is fat. Quite the contrary! Pure oil is not only healthy, but also fights certain diseases. Often, all the body needs is oil to properly transport and absorb certain nutrients.

Oil also helps with weight loss. I told that as a child we took pure oil as a laxative and how it worked. In Cameroon, they "drink" oil, they say. But people there are much slimmer and more muscular than people here in Europe. I cook for my whole family in Germany with plenty of oil.

Oil is a remedy

Good vegetable oil (coconut oil, palm oil, peanut oil, olive oil, rapeseed oil also sunflower oil) helps the stomach to do its job, it cleanses the intestines and helps to eliminate bad substances, toxins, fats and garbage from the body, it is antibacterial, protects against infections, strengthens the immune system, helps to build muscles, strengthens the nerves, lets us absorb vital substances well. Palm oil, for example, is very good for nausea or poisoning. In Africa, palm oil is also used to treat smoke and gas poisoning. Pregnant women often consume raw palm oil so that they don't get sick and it helps the child to develop well. I was told that it is important for pregnant women to consume palm oil all the time, especially just before giving birth, because it makes the birth easier. I noticed that women in Cameroon are taking more and more "modern" oils as a result of industry advertising and also have more difficult births than women used to. "Coincidental" coincidence?

Oil helps a good digestion and contributes to the fact that the food tastes delicious and that you eat less. You are more quickly satiated and thus you also lose weight. Oil can even reduce bad cholesterol.

Bad vegetable oils, bad animal oils and fats full of chemicals are a danger to the body. Butter, cream and the like should be consumed with great caution because the animals that give us these products are also pumped full of chemicals. These chemical additives automatically end up in the products of these animals and poison us when we consume them.

A 2010 report in *Men's Health* magazine said the following: *Fats have important roles in the body. They form a protective component of cell membranes, serve as transporters for fat-soluble vitamins, can be stored in the body as depot fat and tapped when energy is needed. There are saturated, monounsaturated and polyunsaturated fatty acids. The polyunsaturated ones should not be missing from your diet. "The balance of omega-3 and omega-6 fatty acids is important," says nutritionist and book author Ulrike Gonder (*Fett!*, Hirzel-Verlag, around 17 euros). "Omega-6 fatty acids you take up automatically* *with the food in sufficient measure. But to also get a corresponding amount of omega-3 fatty acids, you need to put sea fish, walnuts, flaxseed and rapeseed oil on the menu more often." Omega-3 fatty acids boost fat burning and heat release and have vasodilatory and blood pressure-lowering effects.*

I would say that healthy and chemical-free oils are healthy for the body and unhealthy oils are also unhealthy and dangerous for the body. But the fact is that our cells, membranes and organs need oil.

Oil causes the cells to remain younger, more stable and less susceptible to destruction by free radicals. Oil also fights cancer and its development. Especially against breast cancer, oil is very important. Is it a coincidence that many women who have breast cancer don't use enough oil in their cooking? I have had this knowledge since I was an apprentice almost 40 years ago. One of the best protectors against breast cancer is oil, my teachers used to say and palm oil and peanut oil in particular would be very important. They also contain many phenolic compounds that are strong antioxidants. They should also help the body to better tolerate conventional medical therapy.

Good oils, especially if they are not mixed with chemicals, are: Hemp oil, macadamia oil, sesame oil, pumpkin seed oil, walnut oil, almond oil, pecan oil, flaxseed oil, avocado oil, coconut oil, palm oil, peanut oil.

Along with carbohydrates and proteins, fats are one of the three basic nutrients.

Unsaturated fats are considered "good" fats, which are divided into monounsaturated and polyunsaturated fats. Only the omega-6 fatty acid and the omega-3 fatty acid must be supplied with food, which is why they are also called essential fatty acids.

Omega-6 fatty acids are responsible, for example, for growth, wound healing or protection against infection. Omega-3 fatty acids are found in salmon, tuna, herring, mackerel and tofu, and omega-6 fatty acids in sunflower, safflower, corn and soybean oil.

Polyunsaturated fats are found, for example, in fatty fish such as salmon, herring and mackerel and in vegetable oils.

Monounsaturated fats are found, for example, in olive oil, rapeseed oil or nuts. They play an important role in blood clotting and in the transmission of nerve messages and improve the balance of cholesterol levels.

Obesity and its consequences are not caused by too much fat intake in the diet, but by bad fats.

C3.6 Natural antibiotics, natural foods that are antibacterial and act like antibiotics

Animals in nature also sometimes have chronic infections, but they cure themselves without any industrial antibiotics, only with herbal remedies.

People around the world swallow several thousand tons of chemical antibiotics every year. Often, these are superfluous and they do not even help properly with all diseases. These chemicals can even cause other diseases. Even though the effectiveness of antibiotics for many diseases is lifesaving and not in question, we can still do without them in many cases and turn to nature. Nature has provided for mankind and given us natural remedies, some of which work better than the drugs from the laboratory, which sometimes cost billions.

Essential oils are ingredients of numerous foods and the basis of antibiotic-active herbal remedies.

Here are some natural foods that can inhibit the growth of other microorganisms or even kill them:

- Moringa, a miracle cure, a remedy for everything
- Ginger
- Onion
- Garlic
- Hot palm oil
- Palm kernels, ground
- Hemp agrimony
- Cranberries
- Thyme
- Yarrow
- Myrtle
- Nasturtium
- Umckaloabo root
- South Afriacn geranium
- Turmeric
- Propolis
- Honey
- Horseradish
- Sage
- Green mango
- Green papaya

- Hot chili peppers and their leaves
- Okra

C3.7 Ginger, onion, garlic: Three magical, hypogean, secret weapons for health, against obesity and anti-cancer

The mixture of ginger, garlic and onion is a secret weapon par excellence against cancer. When cooking, it is very advisable to at least use these three spices, fresh. The food then not only tastes good, but it is also healthy and cures or prevents diseases.

Having these three roots in your food constantly in sufficient quantities prevents cancer!

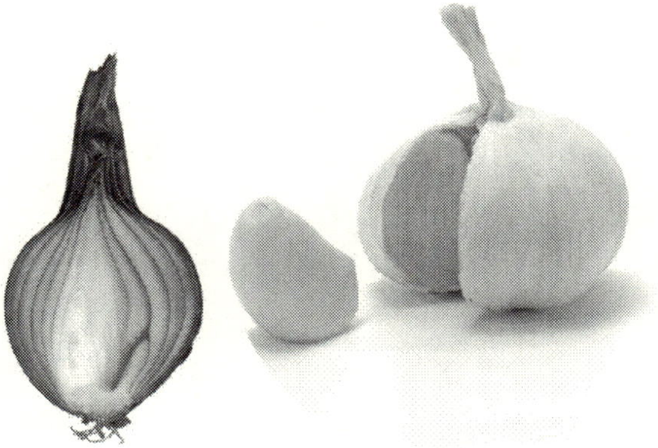

Onions stimulate the digestive glands and build the intestinal flora. Garlic is very important for the body. Garlic can do a lot, people knew this thousands of years ago. In Africa, garlic is even called a "doping agent". Mixed with onion and ginger, it helps very well to lose weight.

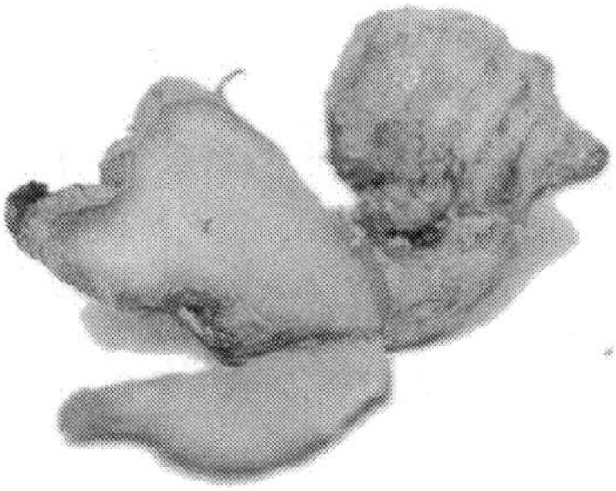

In West Africa and the Caribbean, people have been using the healthy power of ginger for more than 3000 years, especially in West Africa. It was only a few years ago that modern medicine discovered the power of ginger, but the pharmaceutical industry is the winner of this knowledge and not the people who are not properly and clearly explained how and what they can achieve with ginger.

The ginger is slightly spicy when eaten fresh and very spicy in food. Ginger is also an excellent source of potent phytochemicals. The ginger roots stimulate the appetite and circulation, strengthen the stomach and promote digestion, they are antibacterial, promote blood circulation, increase the production of bile, break down fat in the body, promote the desire for sex, are a powerful anti-cold agent, anti-cancer agent and much more. I haven't had a cold since I started eating ginger all the time. No matter if people around me have colds or not. As soon as the outbreak of the common cold starts, I eat raw ginger all the time and just leave it in my mouth like candy and get protected by it.

Many studies show the anti-cancer effect of these three roots. All three contain many antioxidants and other substances that effectively protect against cancer. The naturopaths I met in Cameroon said that these three spices, together with hot chili peppers, are particularly effective in protecting against cancer or against its rapid development in the long term. Scientific studies show that they inhibit tumor growth, and in doing so, they attack only the diseased cells. Healthy cells are not attacked, they are even protected. These roots are very suitable against breast, liver, lung, colon, prostate and stomach cancer.

Those who eat with the three spices are said to significantly reduce the risk of cancer. In Cameroon, these three roots are used as standard for many dishes. The healing effect also has to do with the quantity. The more the better.

Ginger has arrived in Western culture, but very few people really cook with it on a regular basis. If they do cook with it once, they only take a small piece, just a clove or two of garlic and a small onion. And very rarely all three together. That hardly has any effect. The quantity also makes the healing power. Also, ginger tea works only the higher the concentration of ginger in the tea. For this, these spices should always be used fresh. Ginger best in organic quality to use with its skin. In Africa, they say that in the skin are many healing substances.

Mixing these three spices that come from the ground into the good oil when cooking will later help the body process the majority of the fats in a healthy way without depositing them as fat deposits.

In addition, these three spices fight obesity (also a source of cancer) and mental illnesses, such as depression, anxiety, stress and more.

C3.8 Bitter foods and substances are good for our health and help to lose weight, bitter makes fit and slim

Bitter makes you healthy and slim, my mother said every time we ate a Cameroonian dish called "dolet". This dish is prepared with bitter vegetables. We also drank the juices of this vegetable to "cleanse the belly", as it was usually said. In the cold season we were advised to eat foods with bitter substances, they would strengthen the immune system.

Drink and eat bitter not only for the figure, but also for health. The original diet of man was not sweet and salty. It included a variety of foods containing bitter substances: spices, vegetables (roots and leafy vegetables) and wild plants.

When I completed my teaching in Cameroon about nature and its many ways to help people, I was told that substances that are very important for the body as well as toxins can only be absorbed or excreted well if our digestion works properly. Only when digestion is functioning optimally, weight loss can also be successful and healthy in the long term. Bitter foods help a good digestion.

Bitter foods, such as chicory, stimulate the metabolism and promote digestion due to the bitter substances they contain. "It [chicory] stimulates the formation of gastric juice and pancreatic juice and thus the utilization of food" says a scientist, confirming the ancient knowledge from Africa that has existed for thousands of years.

Bitter substances and foods reduce food cravings. In addition, one has a faster feeling of satiety and eats less.

Since bitter foods reduce the desire for sweet and unhealthy foods and have few calories themselves, they help the body accumulate less fat and therefore you lose weight.

The following vegetables and herbs contain large amounts of bitter substances:

- Artichoke
- Dandelion
- Valerian
- Chicory
- Kohlrabi
- Radicchio
- Mugwort
- Hops (wild hops)
- Endive
- Brussels sprouts
- Broccoli
- Grapefruit
- Olives
- Cocoa (pure without sugar)
- Peppermint
- Arugula

With these foods you can prepare great dishes and drinks!

C3.8 Alkaline food, alkaline diet: The basis for a healthy, balanced and strong body and for the elimination of diseases.

The alkaline diet provides the person with easily absorbable alkaline minerals and all the nutrients and vital substances that the body needs to find its healthy balance. At the same time, the alkaline diet spares the person from all those acidic metabolic residues that are produced in the body during the usual diet. In this way, the acid-alkaline balance is harmonized so that the correct and healthy pH level can re-emerge in all areas of the body. The result is an active and healthy person full of energy and zest for life.

http://www.zentrum-der-gesundheit.de/basische-ernaehrung-2.html#ixzz3NToymZj3

An alkaline diet prevents hyperacidity of the body. Acidosis is the cause of many chronic diseases and complaints.

a. Tables of alkaline foods and good acid-forming foods

1 Table base forming fruit

Apples	Mangos
Pineapple	Mirabelle plums
Apricots	Nectarines
Avocados	Olives (green, black)
Bananas	Oranges
Pears	Grapefruit

Clementines	Papayas
fresh dates	Peaches
Strawberries	Plums
Figs	Cranberries
Grapefruits	Quince
Blueberries	Greengage
Raspberries	Gooseberries
Honeydew melons	Star fruit
Currants (red, white, black)	Watermelons
Cherries (sour, sweet)	Grapes (white, red)
Kiwis	Lemons
Limes	Plums
Tangerines	

2 Table of alkaline herbs and salads

Basil	Lollo bionda salad
Batavia lettuce	Marjoram
Savory	Horseradish
Borage	Melde (Spanish spinach)
Nettle	Melissa
Watercress	Nutmeg
Chinese cabbage	Cloves
Chicory	Oregano
Chili peppers	Parsley
Dill	Pepper (white, red, black, green)

Curled lettuce	Peppermint
Iceberg lettuce	Allspice (clove pepper)
Endive	Purslane (Postelein)
Lamb's lettuce	Radicchio
Fennel seeds	Cos lettuce
Frisée salad	Rosemary
Garden cress	Arugula (rocket)
Ginger	Saffron
Capers	Sage
Cardamom	Sorrel
Chervil	Chives
Coriander	Black cumin
Lettuce	Celery leaves
Cumin	Spinach, young
Caraway	Thyme
Turmeric (turmeric)	Vanilla
Lettuce	Hyssop
Lovage	Cinnamon
Dandelion	Lemon balm
Lollo rosso lettuce	Zucchini flowers

3 Table of basic shoots and sprouts

Alfalfa sprouts	Lentil sprouts
Amaranth sprouts	Mung bean sprouts
Brown millet sprouts	Broccoli sprouts
Fenugreek sprouts	Radish sprouts
Arugula sprouts	Adzuki bean sprouts

Millet sprouts	Mustard sprouts
Coriander sprouts	Sunflower seed sprouts
Cress	Wheat seedlings
Flaxseed sprouts	Barley seedlings

4 Table of alkaline nuts and alkaline seeds

Almonds	Almond paste
Tigernuts	Chestnuts (sweet chestnuts)

Note: All other nuts/seeds/oilseeds are among the good acid-forming foods. Their acid potential can be further reduced by soaking overnight, i.e. brief germination.

5 Table of alkaline protein and alkaline noodles

Lupin flour	Lupin protein tablets
Alkaline konjac pasta	

6 Good acidifying foods

- Nuts (walnuts, hazelnuts, Brazil nuts, pecans, macadamia nuts, etc.)
- Oil seeds (linseed, sesame, hemp seed, sunflower seeds, pumpkin seeds, poppy seeds, etc. - if the seeds are allowed to germinate, they become alkaline - depending on the germination period).
- Legumes (beans, lentils, chickpeas, dried peas, etc.)

- High quality cocoa powder, preferably raw, and homemade chocolate
- Millet
- Corn (e.g. also polenta, corn pasta) in small quantities
- Pseudocereals (quinoa, amaranth, buckwheat)
- Organic cereals e.g. spelt, kamut or barley in small quantities - ideally as sprouted bread or in sprouted form (if there are no intolerances or health complaints)
- Grain products such as bulgur and couscous in small quantities, but from spelt, not wheat
- In manageable quantities, high-quality animal products from organic farming e.g. organic eggs or fish from organic aquaculture
- High quality organic tofu and high quality fermented soy products such as miso and tempeh
- High quality vegetable protein powders (if there is a protein deficit) such as hemp protein or rice protein.

Source:http://www.zentrum-der-gesundheit.de/saure-und-basische-lebensmittel.html#ixzz3KncqLST6

7 Table of nutritional values of alkaline foods

Food nutritional values (per 100 g)	**kcal**	**kJ**	**BU**	**CH (g)**	**Fat (g)**	**Pro (g)**
Adzuki bean sprouts	52	219	0	3	0,5	3
Alfalfa sprouts (alfalfa, snail clover, eternal clover)	24	100	0	0,4	0,7	4
Top-fermented dark beer	49	208	0,5	3	0	0,5
Amaranth sprouts	31	128	0	2	0,6	4

Food nutritional values (per 100 g)	**kcal**	**kJ**	**BU**	**CH (g)**	**Fat (g)**	**Pro (g)**
Pineapple	55	234	1	12,4	0,2	0,5
Anise tea	9	38	0	0,9	0,4	0,4
Apple	54	228	1	11,4	0,6	0,3
Apple juice, green apple	48	202	1	11,1	0	0,1
Apple juice, red apple	46	193	1	10,3	0,3	0,3
Oranges	42	179	1	8,3	0,2	1
Apricots	43	183	1	8,5	0,1	0,9
Eggplants, Melanzani, Melanzane	17	73	0	2,7	0,2	1,2
Oyster mushrooms	11	45	0	0	0,1	2,3
Avocados	221	909	0	0,4	23,5	1,9
Bananas (strongly alkaline)	88	374	2	20	0,2	1,2
Basil, fresh	46	194	0,5	7,5	0,7	2,4
Batavia lettuce, red lettuce, crisp lettuce	12	50	0	1,5	0,3	0,7
Berliner Weiße with a shot (woodruff, raspberry)	51	214	0,6	7	0	0,3
Pears	55	233	1	12,4	0,3	0,5
Celery, celery stalks	15	65	0	2,2	0,2	1,2
Cauliflower (strongly alkaline)	22	95	0	2,3	0,3	2,5
Fenugreek sprouts	25	1ß3	0	3,1	0,6	1,5
Beans, green (green beans, garden beans, princess beans, kenya beans, bush beans, pole beans, welsh beans, crack beans, Turkish peas, rick beans, string beans, string beans, string beans, runner beans)	33	138	0,5	5,1	0,2	2,4
Beans, white, ripe (strongly alkaline)	260	1102	3	40,1	1,6	21,3
Savory, dried	307	1260	4,5	54	6	7
Borage, dried	189	776	1,5	17	6	14,8

Food nutritional values (per 100 g)	kcal	kJ	BU	CH (g)	Fat (g)	Pro (g)
Boviste (puffball)	18	73	0	1	1	1
French beans, snip beans, snap beans (strongly alkaline)	29	122	0,5	5,1	0,2	1,5
Nettles	70	289	0,5	4,9	5,2	0,7
Nettle tea	3	13	0	0,5	0	0,1
Broccoli	26	111	0	2,5	0,2	3,3
Watercress	20	80	0	2,5	0,3	1,5
Buttermilk, natural	40	170	0,5	4	1	3,5
Mushrooms	16	67	0	0,6	0,3	2,7
Chicory	17	70	0	2,3	0,2	1,3
Chili peppers, green or red	19	81	0	2,9	0,3	1,2
Chinese cabbage	13	54	0	1,3	0,3	1,2
Chlorella algae, dried (green freshwater algae)	428	1798	1,5	18	11	60
Clementines	37	155	1	9	0,3	0,7
Steam beer (top-fermented, but similar to export beer)	65	273	0,5	5	0	0,5
Dates, fresh	56	235	1	12,9,0	0,1	0,5
Dill, fresh	51	216	0,5	6,6	0,9	3,8
Dill, dried	373	1566	0,5	46,3	8,4	25
Iceberg lettuce	13	55	0	1,9	0,3	0,7
Endives, frisée (basic)	10	43	0	0,3	0,2	1,8
Peas, green (strongly alkaline)	81	342	1	12,3	0,5	6,6
Strawberries	32	136	0,5	5,5	0,4	0,8
Espresso, black	2	8	0	0,3	0	0,1
Figs, fresh	61	260	1	12,9	0,5	1,3
Figs, dried (strongly alkaline)	250	1059	5	55	1,3	3,5
Lamb's lettuce, nut lettuce, field lettuce, sun swirl (strongly alkaline)	14	57	0	0,7	0,4	1,8

Food nutritional values (per 100 g)	**kcal**	**kJ**	**BU**	**CH (g)**	**Fat (g)**	**Pro (g)**
Fennel seeds, dried	376	1579	3,5	38	16	17
Fennel tea	10	42	0	1	0,4	0,4
Spring onions	24	104	0	3	0,5	2
Garden lettuce (green lettuce, butter lettuce, butterhead lettuce, lamb's lettuce, lard lettuce, strongly alkaline)	11	48	0	1,1	0,2	1,3
Common giant parasol (Parasol)	14	58	0	0	0,5	2,2
Gomasio, Gomashio (sesame salt)	541	2272	0	0,9	50,6	15,9
Grapefruits	38	161	0,5	7,4	0,1	0,6
Grapefruit juice	47	197	1	10,1	0,1	0,5
Green cardamom, dried	254	1068	5,5	62	7	12
Kale, colewort	37	157	0	3	0,9	4,3
Cucumbers (salad cucumbers, chichinga, strongly alkaline)	12	50	0	1,8	0,1	0,6
Blueberries, , huckleberries, bilberies, forest berries, wild berries, cranberries	36	154	0,5	6,1	0,6	0,6
Raspberries	34	143	0,5	4,8	0,3	1,3
Hokkaido pumpkin, butternut squash, butternut squash	64	270	1	12,6	0,6	1,7
Ginger	69	290	1	12	1	2,5
Ginger tea	2	8	0	0,6	0,1	0,2
Currants, red and white	33	139	0,5	4,8	0,2	1,1
Currants, black	39	168	0,5	6,1	0,2	1,3
Chamomile tea	3	13	0	0,5	0	0,1
Capers (canned)	415	1756	4,5	52	20,2	6

Food nutritional values (per 100 g)	**kcal**	**kJ**	**BU**	**CH (g)**	**Fat (g)**	**Pro (g)**
Mashed potatoes, ready prepared (mashed potatoes, squashed potatoes, strongly alkaline)	74	312	1	12,2	1,9	2
Potatoes, raw (very strongly alkaline)	70	298	1,5	14,8	0,1	2
Sprouts (average values for brown millet sprouts, barley sprouts, coriander seed sprouts, linseed sprouts, radish sprouts, etc.)	26	108	0	2,8	0,4	2,5
Chervil, fresh	51	208	0,5	6,5	0,5	4,5
Cherry, sour (sour cherries)	53	225	1	9,9	0,5	0,9
Cherry, sweet (sweet cherries, heart cherries)	62	265	1	13,2	0,3	0,9
Kiwi	51	215	1	9,1	0,6	1
Celeriac (strongly alkaline)	18	77	0	2,3	0,3	1,6
Kohlrabi, top turnip, turnip cabbage,	24	102	0	3,7	0,1	1,9
Kölsch beer 4.9 % by volume	56	235	0,5	4	0	0,5
Coriander, dried	327	1371	2,5	26	18	12,5
Cress, watercress, garden cress, fresh	33	139	0	2,4	0,7	4,2
Cumin seeds, dried	430	1764	3	35	22,5	18
Caraway seed	375	1576	3	37	15	20
Caraway tea	10	42	0	0,9	0,4	0,5
Pumpkin	24	101	0,5	4,6	0,1	1,1
Pumpkin seeds, grown without shells or peeled	560	2369	1,5	14,2	45,6	24,3

Food nutritional values (per 100 g)	**kcal**	**kJ**	**BU**	**CH (g)**	**Fat (g)**	**Pro (g)**
Turmeric, curcuma, yellow ginger, saffron root, dried (coloring in curry)	366	1536	5	58,5	10	7,8
Leek	24	103	0	3,2	0,3	2,2
Lovage, fresh	51	210	0,5	6	1	4
Limes	31	130	0	1,9	2,4	0,5
Lime blossom tea	3	13	0	0,5	0	0,1
Dandelion leaves (strong alkaline effect)	60	245	1	9,6	1,1	2,5
Marjoram, dried	292	1226	3,5	42	7	12,5
Tangerines (strong alkaline effect)	46	195	1	10,1	0,3	0,7
Almond puree, almond nut puree	648	2720	1	9,5	56,5	19,8
Almonds, sweet, without shell	599	2507	0,5	3,7	54,1	18,7
Mango	57	243	1	12,5	0,5	0,6
Chard, leaf chard, cut chard, ribbed chard, stemmed chard, cabbage stem, turnip stem	14	59	0	0,7	0,3	2,1
Horseradish, freshly grated	67	281	1	12,2	0,5	2,9
Melde, garden melde (Spanish spinach)	24	99	0	2,9	0,3	2,1
Mini peppers, snack peppers (sweet peppers, bell peppers)	37	154	0,5	6,4	0,5	1,4
Mirabelle plums	63	269	1,5	14	0,2	0,7
Poppy seed	477	1976	0,5	4,2	42,2	20,2
Carrots	25	108	0,5	4,8	0,2	1
Whey, sour (milk serum)	21	89	0,5	4,2	0,2	0,6
Whey, sweet (milk serum)	25	106	0,5	4,7	0,2	0,8
Morels (soaked)	10	40	0	0	0,3	1,7

Food nutritional values (per 100 g)	kcal	kJ	BU	CH (g)	Fat (g)	Pro (g)
Judas ear, elderberry mushrooms, jelly ear (soaked)	10	40	0	0	0,3	1,7
Mung bean sprouts, golden gram sprouts	24	99	0,5	2	0,2	3,2
Nutmeg, dried	548	2303	4	45	36,5	5,8
Nectarines	42	180	1	9	0,1	1,4
Baked potatoes (strongly alkaline)	111	467	1,5	16	4	2
Okra fruit, "okra", fresh	19	81	0	2,2	0,2	2
Olives, green, marinated	138	569	0	1,8	13,9	1,4
Olives, black, marinated	135	555	0	1,5	13,8	1,1
Orange juice (OJ)	44	185	1	9	0,2	0,7
Oregano, rye brome, wild thyme, dried	349	1465	4	50	10,5	11
Papaya	12	53	0	2,4	0,1	0,5
Peppers, yellow (bell peppers, paprika pods)	28	117	0,5	4,9	0,3	1,2
Peppers, green (bell peppers, paprika pods)	20	86	0	2,9	0,3	1,2
Peppers, red (bell peppers, paprika pods)	33	141	0,5	6,4	0,4	1
Parsnip, parsnip (raw)	58	245	1	12	0,2	0,7
Boiled jacket potatoes, mashed potatoes (strongly alkaline)	70	298	1,5	14,8	0,1	2
Parsley (leaves), fresh	50	214	0,5	7,4	0,4	4,4
Parsley (root), fresh	41	174	0,5	6	0,5	2,9
Pepper, black, dried (black pepper)	278	1166	4,5	51,9	3,3	11
Pepper, white, dried (white pepper)	278	1166	4,5	51,9	3,3	11
Peppermint (fresh)	44	185	0,5	5,5	0,5	4
Peppermint tea	3	13	0	0,5	0	0,1

Food nutritional values (per 100 g)	**kcal**	**kJ**	**BU**	**CH (g)**	**Fat (g)**	**Pro (g)**
Peppers, hot peppers	20	83	0	0,7	0,6	2,9
Chanterelles	11	47	0	0,2	0,5	1,5
Chanterelles, dried	93	391	0	1,8	2,2	16,5
Peaches	41	176	1	8,9	0,1	0,8
Plums	48	205	1	10,2	0,2	0,6
Allspice, dried (clove pepper)	314	1318	4	50	9	6
Leek	24	103	0	3,2	0,3	2,2
Purslane,Indian lettuce, Cuban spinach, winter purslane, spring beauty	29	119	0,5	4,5	0,4	1,6
Cranberries	35	148	0,5	6,2	0,5	0,3
Quince, apple quince, pear quince	39	165	0,5	6,9	1	0,4
Radicchio (lollo rosso)	13	53	0	1,5	0,2	1,2
Radish	14	58	0	2,2	0,1	1
Greengage	45	187	1	10,2	0,2	0,2
Radish (strong alkaline effect)	13	57	0	1,9	0,2	1
Romaine lettuce, cos lettuce	16	67	0	1,8	0,2	1,6
Romanesco (cauliflower style)	30	127	0	4,5	0,5	1,7
Raisins (strongly alkalizing)	277	1178	6	63,9	0,6	2,5
Rosemary, fresh	60	252	1	10	2	0
Beet (beetroot)	41	175	0	8,6	0,1	1,5
Red cabbage, blue cabbage	22	92	0	3,5	0,2	1,5
Arugula, curled lettuce, rocket	11	48	0	1,1	0,2	1,3
Saffron, dried	356	1496	5	61,5	6	11,5
Sage spice, dried	334	1403	3,5	43	12	11
Sage, fresh	87	365	1	12	3,2	1,9
Sage tea	9	38	0	0,9	0,4	0,4
Boiled potatoes, cooked (strongly alkaline)	70	298	1,5	15,4	0,1	1,8

Food nutritional values (per 100 g)	**kcal**	**kJ**	**BU**	**CH (g)**	**Fat (g)**	**Pro (g)**
Sorrel (strong alkaline effect)	22	92	0	2	0,4	2,4
Shallots (scallions, spring onions)	77	325	1,5	16,1	0,1	2,5
Chives, fresh	27	114	0	1,6	0,7	3,6
Black salsify	16	66	0	1,6	0,4	1,4
Seaweed (sea algae)	54	228	1	12	0,5	1,8
Seaweed, dried (marine algae)	278	1166	5	55	2	8
Sesame paste (tahina, tahini sesame puree, sesame puree)	638	2680	0	1	60	18,1
Sesame seeds	598	2472	0	1	58	18,2
Shitake, dried	336	1411	4,5	53	3,5	20,5
Soybeans, ripe	323	1350	0,5	6,3	18,1	33,7
Soy flakes	360	1512	0,5	4	20	37,5
Soy bran	129	541	0,5	7	4	15
Soy flour, full fat (soy flour)	347	1449	0	3,1	20,6	37,3
Soy milk	36	151	0	0,7	1,9	3,6
Soy cream	184	773	0	2	18	2
Soybean sprouts	50	211	0,5	4,7	1	5,5
Asparagus (strong alkaline effect)	18	77	0	2,2	0,2	1,9
Spinach, leaf spinach (strongly alkaline)	15	64	0	0,6	0,3	2,5
Spirulina, dried (algae in alkaline inland waters, antiviral against Epstein-Barr virus).	376	1579	0	3	12	60
Pointed cabbage (sugar loaf)	23	97	0	2,7	0,4	2
Gooseberries	37	158	0,5	7,1	0,2	0,8
Porcini (cep, summer bolete)	20	85	0	0,5	0,4	3,6
Porcini, dried (cep, summer bolete)	124	523	0,5	4,1	3,2	19,7
Star fruit, carambola (oxalic acid)	44	185	1	9,5	0,3	0,5

Food nutritional values (per 100 g)	**kcal**	**kJ**	**BU**	**CH (g)**	**Fat (g)**	**Pro (g)**
Turnip greens, raw, rapini turnip greens	28	116	0	2,8	0,6	2,5
Sweet potatoes	111	467	2	24,1	0,6	1,6
Tea, green, without sugar (green tea)	0	2	0	0,1	0	0
Tea, herbal tea	3	13	0	0,5	0	0,1
Tea, mate green / roasted	0	2	0	0	0	0,1
Tea, white, without sugar (white tea)	0	2	0	0,1	0	0
Thyme, dried	292	1227	4	45	7,5	9
Thyme tea	3	13	0	0,5	0	0,1
Tomatoes, strained tomatoes (strongly alkaline)	19	79	0	2,7	0,2	1,2
Tomato juice	17	71	0	2,9	0,1	0,8
Truffles, truffle mushrooms	40	167	0	3	1	4,3
Vanilla beans (orchid type), dried	278	1166	5	56,1	3,3	4
Wakame (seaweed for miso) Attention: about 15 mg iodine per 100 gram!	55	229	1	9	1	2
Watermelons	37	159	1	8,3	0,2	0,6
Grapes, red	74	312	1,5	17	0,3	0,7
Grapes, white	67	286	1,5	16,1	0,3	0,7
White turnips	24	103	0	4,6	0,2	1
White cabbage	25	104	0	4,1	0,2	1,4
Wheat beer	52	222	0,5	3	0	0,3
Wheat beer non-alcoholic	24	101	0,5	5,4	0	0,4
Savoy cabbage (strongly alkaline)	25	107	0	2,4	0,4	3
Hyssop leaves	30	126	0	2,9	0,6	3
Cinnamon sticks, cinnamon powder	283	1189	5	57	3,5	4

Food nutritional values (per 100 g)	**kcal**	**kJ**	**BU**	**CH (g)**	**Fat (g)**	**Pro (g)**
Lemons	35	151	0,5	3,2	0,6	0,7
Lemon balm, fresh	50	205	0,5	5,5	1	4,2
Lemon juice	26	109	0	2,4	0,1	0,4
Zucchini	18	76	0	2	0,4	1,6
Sugar melons, honeydew melons	54	230	1	12,4	0,1	0,9
Plums, damsons, plums (plum type)	40	168	1	8,9	0,1	0,6
Onions, red onions (strong alkaline)	28	117	0	4,9	0,3	1,3

Source: http://www.lebensmittel-tabelle.de/basische-lebensmittel.html

Legend:

kcal = kilocalories
kJ = kilojoules
BU = bread units (rounded)
CH (g) = carbohydrates contained in grams
Fat (g) = fat contained in grams
Pro (g) = proteins contained in grams
1g fat = 9.3 kcal
1g Pro = 4.2 kcal
1g CH = 4.1 kcal
1g alcohol = 7.0 kcal
1g org. acid = 3.0 kcal

C3.9 Some tropical foods with strong healing power

C3.9.1 Moringa tree (Moringa oleifera) - The miracle tree

The most nutrient-rich plant in the world, known in Cameroon as "mother's best friend" or "tree of life," cures many diseases and cancer. I will report on this in more detail in the book "Healthy and Vital: Healing Power from the tropics".

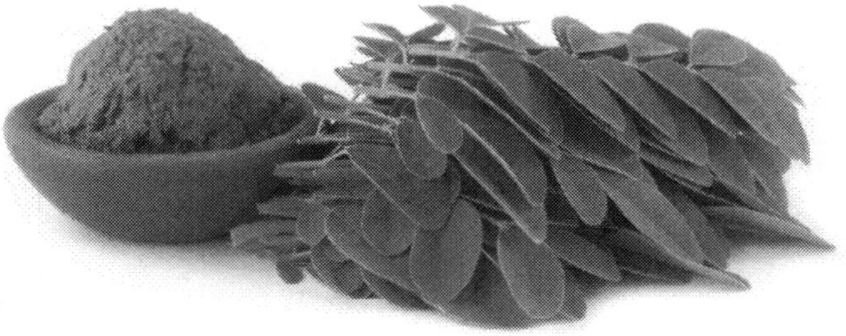

This tree seems to be one of the most valuable plants and food for our health and can cure hundreds of diseases. It was only when I visited natural medicine practitioners in Cameroon for my book on cancer that I learned about this plant, which has been used successfully in natural medicine for centuries to cure chronic diseases and infections.

In Cameroon, almost everything on this tree is eaten (leaves, bark, seeds, flowers, pods, etc.). It took me a long time to learn the scientific name of this plant. In Cameroon, they just call it "do not die plant, mother's best friend, tree of life," etc. I knew the tree was a miracle tree without knowing exactly why. Only when I wanted to know more about it and intensively studied all the plants in Cameroon, I found the name and was not surprised that there is already scientific literature and studies about it worldwide. In Cameroon, moringa is used to treat many diseases such as anemia, cancer, maternal and infant mortality, diabetes, skin diseases, inflammation, wound healing, cardiovascular diseases, rheumatism, dementia, Parkinson's disease, AIDS, eye and dental diseases, impotence, bronchitis, fever, brittle bones, malnutrition, diarrhea, stomach pain, fungal infections, diseased intestinal flora and many more.

Furthermore, Moringa can be used to purify water by destroying 90% to 99% of bacteria. Its seeds contain 40% oil. This oil is more valuable than olive oil. Moringa is a top organic feed for animals and an excellent fertilizer.

It has an enormously high **content of nutrients, vitamins and minerals** and has an extreme and exceptional antioxidant potential.

"The combination and composition of **vital substances** is very concentrated, balanced and unique among all known plants" can be read on http://www.moringafarm.eu/. According to this page, the moringa tree contains:

14 vitamins

13 minerals

8 essential amino acids

10 non-essential amino acids

Omega-3, -6 and -9 fatty acids

secondary phytochemicals

over 46 antioxidants

zeatin, salvestrols and chlorophyll

The page continues to read:

...Comparison results of moringa leaf powder to 1058 foods, based on the Nutrition Information System of the University of Hohenheim.

- 100 grams of leaf powder from Moringa oleifera contain in comparison:
- 17 x as much calcium as 3.5% cow's milk
- 1.3 x more essential amino acids than eggs
- 6 x more alpha-linolenic acid than linoleic acid
- 1.9 x more fiber than whole wheat
- 8.8 x more iron than a beef fillet (loin)
- 6 x more heart-protecting polyphenols than red wine
- 4.7 x more folic acid than beef liver
- 4.5 x more vitamin E than wheat sprouts
- 1.5 x more zinc than a pork cutlet
- about as much vitamin C as a fruit salad
- 7 x more magnesium than shrimp
- 37 x more antioxidant effect than grapes
- 6.9 x more vitamin B1 and B2 than yeast
- 3 x more potassium than bananas
- up to 3 x more eye-protective lutein than kale
- 4 x more vitamin A than carrots
- very high levels of unsaturated fatty acids (omega 3, 6 and 9)
- furthermore, very large amounts of natural chlorophyll

C3.9.2 Okra, another miracle (healing) food

The okra is one of the oldest vegetable plants. It is a vegetable plant native to the highlands of East Africa, from Ethiopia, which is eaten throughout Africa. The name "okra" comes from the Ibo language in Nigeria. The okra becomes slimy when cooked and is eaten as a sauce with all carbohydrates or simply as a salad.

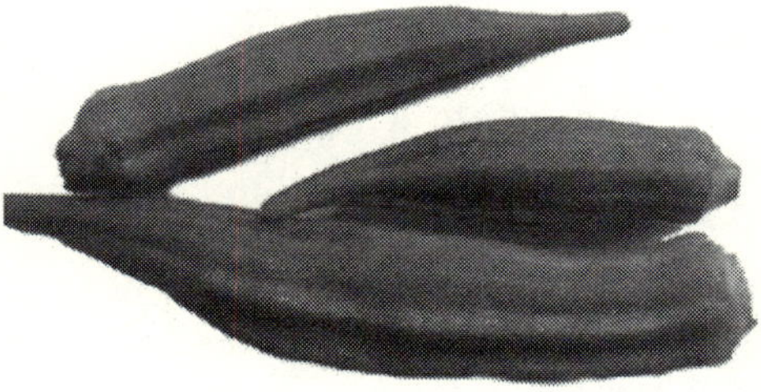

Okra is the source of many vitamins and minerals.

Anyone who regularly eats okra is obviously doing their intestines a big favor. The green vegetable from Africa is on the advance to Europe. It not only proves itself as a versatile ingredient in the kitchen, but also unfolds its health-promoting powers as a valued medicinal plant.

Source: www.zentrum-der-gesundheit.de

Nutritional values okra* per 100g / daily requirement of an adult

Energy: 81 kJ / 19 kcal
Dietary fiber: 4.9 g
Fat: 0.2 g

Carbohydrates: 2.2 g
Protein: 2.1 g

Beta-carotene: 394 µg / 800 µg
Vitamin C: 36 mg / 60 mg
Magnesium: 38 mg / 250-500 mg
Calcium:64 mg / 800 mg
Iron: 653 µg / 15 mg
Phosphorus: 75 mg / 1000 mg

* Nutritional information for okra according to DGE (German Nutrition Society).

In addition, vitamins B2, B3, B6, B9, vitamin K, and copper.

In Africa, okra is more than a normal food, it is a medicine, an antioxidant.

Okra is anti-inflammatory, lowers cholesterol and helps with intestinal problems, diabetes, inflammation of the mouth and throat, asthma, colds, fever, impotence, dry vagina, listlessness, painful menstruation, depression, weak heart muscle and much more.

Certain mixtures with okra act like viagra and strengthen potency.

The pharmaceutical industry uses the mucilage of okra to produce medicines for colds and chest pains.

C3.9.3 Djansang, medicinal herb from Cameroon

Djansang or njangsa is a yellow seed from the green, kidney-shaped fruit of a tree in the rainforest of Africa. It is food and medicine at the same time.

The United States Department of Agriculture (USDA) and the U.S. National Institute of Food and Agriculture (NIFA) prompted a study of this seed in 2013 that shows how important it is.

Njangsa seed oil is rich in polyunsaturated fatty acids and djansang is rich in calcium, magnesium, iron, chlorine, phosphorus, potassium. Like the seed, the oil contains vitamin E and A, proteins, carbohydrates. The oil has a natural healing and soothing effect for skin burns. It also provides protection against sunburn. Cosmetic companies have recognized the value of this oil and use it in numerous creams. Women in Cameroon use this oil to have elastic and wrinkle-free skin.

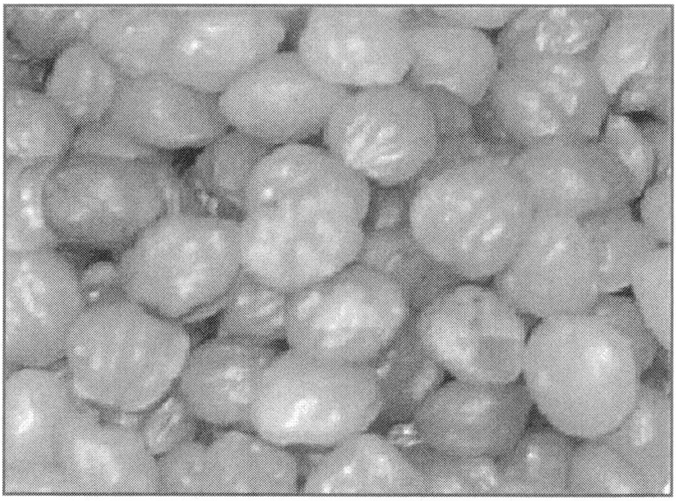

Roasted and ground into a paste, the seeds are also used to make a delicious sauce reminiscent of peanut sauce. But you can also puree the seeds just like that and refine sauces with them.

The leaves and bark of djansang are used to cure or prevent many diseases: cough, malaria, yellow fever, stomach pain, diarrhea, rheumatism, insomnia, cardiovascular diseases, inflammation in body. Eye inflammations and infertility in women. It is a very powerful antioxidant against free radicals.

Djansang is also used as a natural birth control pill, it improves the quality of breast milk and strengthens sexual desire and potency in both women and men.

Djansang contains lupeol, which is a secondary plant compound that belongs to the pentacyclic triterpenes and also belongs to the group of alcohols. Lupeol has been known for more than a hundred years and is of interest to medical researchers as a potentially readily available antimalarial and anticancer agent with low toxicity. It is believed to inhibit the growth of tumor cells. Due to the lupeol, djansang also has an antimicrobial effect.

Djangsang seeds can be bought in most Afro stores or on the Internet. Beware of powder, it often contains admixtures. The best way is to buy the seeds and mash them yourself. Then add a little olive oil, let it stand for a few days and then filter it. The oil is also used for the skin. You will see amazing results after some time.

C3.9.4 Palm oil, better than many anti-cancer drugs?

Palm oil, also called palm fat, is extracted from the pulp of the palm fruit.

The bad reputation of palm oil is not understandable, because this oil has been the most important oil in many countries in Africa and elsewhere for thousands of years. It is portrayed as a bad oil because of its high saturated fat content. Once again, this is a serious misconception. (Coconut oil is also very high in saturated acid, but is considered a "good oil" in Western nations.) The saturated fatty acids are not alone and this makes an enormous difference.

Many studies in Africa on people who traditionally eat a diet largely based on palm oil have disproved the disease-causing effect attributed to saturated fatty acids: Cardiovascular disease was virtually unheard of in those studied, as it was in people who eat a lot of coconut oil. Moreover, these people are much slimmer and more muscular than inhabitants of Western countries.

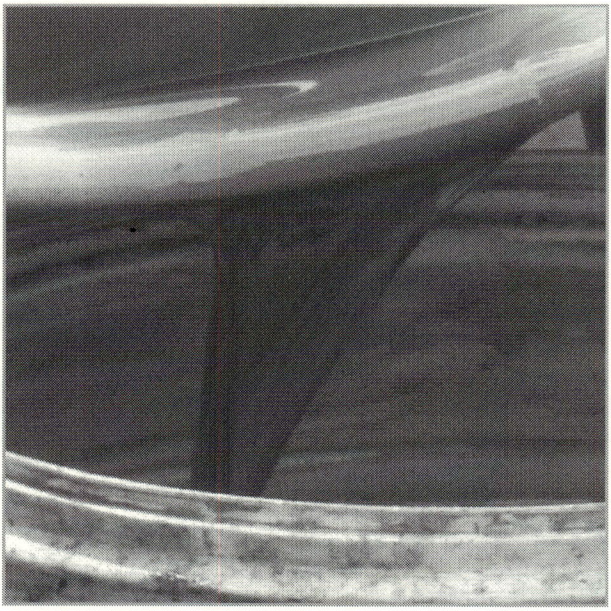

While refined palm oil, like almost all refined oils, is considered unhealthy, natural palm oil is more than a food: it's a medicine. Nutrition experts only see the content of fatty acids and sound the alarm. They forget that saturated oil is not evil per se, no, it depends on the whole composition of this oil, which is much more important. And this composition of substances is almost perfect in palm oil, making it an excellent agent against the growth of cancerous tumors. It helps against cardiovascular diseases, Alzheimer's disease, stroke. It has also been proven that it permanently lowers the dangerous LDL cholesterol level.

"Red palm oil is considered a true nutrient pool. Besides its excellent fatty acid composition, it also contains phytosterols, flavonoids, phenolic acids, glycolipids, vitamin K, Q-10 and squalene. In addition, it is THE source of vitamin E, as it has all four tocotrienols, whose tremendous antioxidant activity is up to 60 times higher than that of normal vitamin E. Combined with its beta-carotene, alpha-carotene, lycopene, as well as another 20 carotenes, it is an excellent antioxidant food that protects teeth and gums from free radical attack." According to www.zentrum-der-gesundheit.de.

In Africa, palm oil is not only used to cook, but also to heal. So as children, we were lotioned with palm oil for skin problems, licked palm oil for stomach aches and pains. The oil was used to fight cellulite. For skin burns, the wound was anointed with palm oil. Many natural medicine practitioners also used palm oil to cure chronic diseases, even cancer. It is supposed to be particularly good against prostate and breast cancer because it is also supposed to fight the metastases, better than chemotherapy, my teacher stated. Palm oil is already used in the treatment of breast cancer. It is also used to fight skin cancer.

Studies also show that palm oil prevents thrombosis by dissolving the deposits in the arteries.

The bad reputation of palm oil also has to do with what others call the destruction of forests. But the right fight would be to go against the Western corporations, the pharmaceutical and food industry, for which the great part of this oil is produced. Many medicines, foods, cosmetic products that we use, that save us, make us full and more beautiful contain palm oil. A very simple logic would have been not to put this oil, since it is so "bad", in medicines, right? It is quite frightening how false information is spread to influence people, while this oil is richer in, for example, important vitamin E than olive oil, which also contains saturated fatty acids.

Palm oil and breast cancer

Palm oil is said to fight breast cancer.

Palm oil is very efficient against breast cancer, better than the drug docetaxel, according to a study by Li Ka Shing of the Faculty of Medicine of Hong Kong University and the Australian Centre for Prostate Cancer Research. The fruit of the oil palm is very rich in tocotrienol. Experiments in the laboratory have shown that this natural compound is more powerful than docetaxel, a drug used in chemotherapy to treat breast cancer. The researchers discovered that tocotrienol has an anti-cancer effect. It fights metastases without the side effects of chemotherapy, which also attacks healthy cells. This confirms the findings of African natural medicine, which has been treating cancer with palm oil for many years.

C3.9.5 Coconut oil and coconut

Coconut oil is one of the most valuable foods because of its many positive effects on health. It is not only for cooking, but also a medicine for the body, skin, hair, etc. and it stimulates digestion. It has antibacterial, antiviral, antifungal and antiparasitic effects. Because of the lauric acid it contains, it kills bacteria, viruses and fungi. Coconut oil inhibits chronic inflammation, cleanses the intestinal flora and strengthens the immune system. Coconut oil also contains many medium-chain triglycerides and can thus be used very well against Alzheimer's disease.

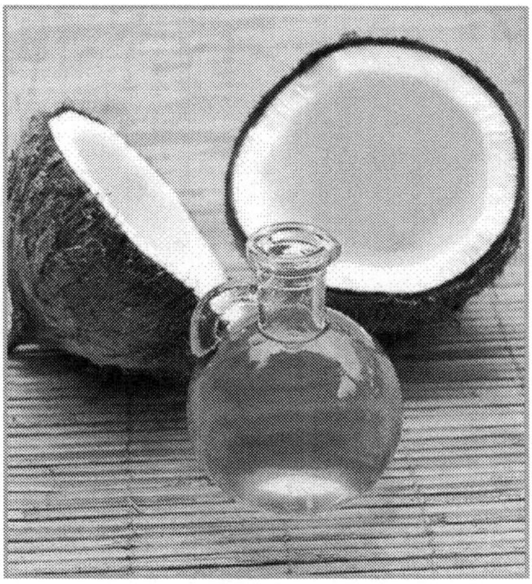

Coconut also prevents cancer; in Cameroon coconut is recommended for men to keep their prostate healthy and for women to keep their breasts healthy. Numerous scientific studies confirm the healing properties of coconut oil against cancer and even against its development. There are reported cases where women with breast cancer became healthier by consuming coconut oil daily. It was said that the metastases were stopped and the cancer receded.

Coconut oil can reduce obesity, according to a Brazilian study published in the journal *Lipids in* 2009. Women who consumed 30 milliliters of coconut oil daily for 12 weeks lost a noticeable amount of weight. In contrast, women in the comparison group who consumed the same amount of soybean oil during the same period did not lose any weight.

Coconut is known for its antibacterial, antioxidant, antiparasitic, blood sugar-lowering and immunostimulant properties. It contains many vitamins, minerals and trace elements and provides the body with calcium, magnesium, phosphorus, iron, sodium, selenium, iodine, zinc, fluorine and manganese, among others.

Coconut is also considered to have anti-stress and anti-osteoporosis effects. It prevents water retention and helps in weight loss. It is also a good cleanser for the body and very healthy for Parkinson's and Alzheimer's disease. Pregnant women should consume coconut, it is an excellent fruit for mother and child because it is a great help during pregnancy with its nutrients, vitamins and energy.

Especially for diabetics, coconut is very healthy. The medium-length fatty acids it contains lower insulin resistance and they stimulate the pancreas to produce more insulin.

Coconut milk strengthens the cardiovascular system, it can rid the kidneys of harmful substances and it protects against vomiting, flatulence and urological complaints. Coconut milk has similar properties to breast milk and is recommended for children because of the vitamin C it contains, natural sugar and many minerals.

C3.9.6 Pineapple: good mood fruit, anti-cancer fruit, ideal for brain and an antidepressant.

A super food for the psyche and to combat hyperacidity of the body and many diseases.

The pineapple is not only a delicious fruit, it is a powerful remedy that provides our body with important minerals and trace elements such as magnesium, calcium, phosphorus, potassium, iron, manganese, zinc and iodine. The tropical good mood fruit is also a supplier of important vitamins, including beta-carotene (pro-vitamin A), biotin, vitamin C, vitamin E, riboflavin, thiamin, niacin, and many more. Fresh pineapple juice has a very positive effect on fever.

Pineapple is an ideal fruit to play an important role in the deacidification of the body, because it has a very alkaline effect due to its minerals.

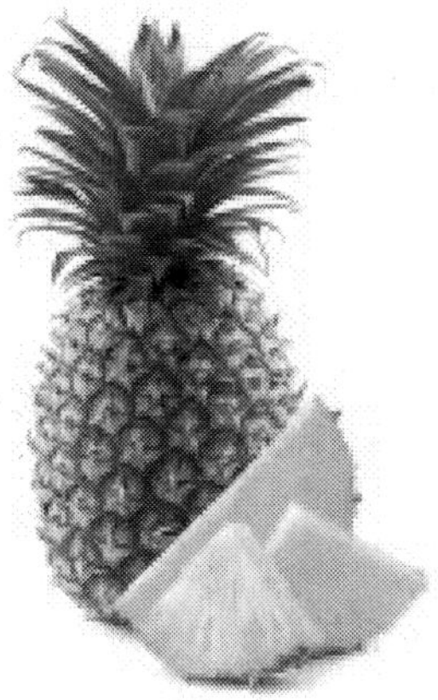

Pineapple also works wonders for the psyche and in stressful situations, it puts you in a good mood, is good for the brain and skin and promotes the desire for sex. It contains natural vanillin and the neurotransmitter serotonin and its precursor tryptophan, which stimulate good mood, relaxation and feelings of satisfaction, curb food cravings, counteract anger, restlessness, aggressiveness, anxiety and nervousness and also have a euphoric and eroticizing effect.

Tryptophan is even offered as an antidepressant in the USA, but as a mild sleeping pill and sedative in Germany. It has been found that people who have depression have very low serotonin levels.

Pineapple and cancer

Pineapple is an antioxidant and successfully prevents inflammation in the body, protecting it from chronic diseases. Pineapple contains the enzyme bromelain. This can also help against cancer. A study published in the journal *Cancer Letter* proves this effect. The researchers were able to prove that bromelain is effective and helpful in the prevention of cancer and tumor formation. It is anti-inflammatory and can activate immune cells, preventing them from dying. It seems, according to studies, that bromelain can kill cancer cells even without other therapy.

In Africa, pineapple is also used for skin problems, injuries, internal and external inflammation, scarlet fever, bladder problems, kidney inflammation and pain, stomach and digestive problems, muscle tension and cramps, sore throat, colds, potency problems, listlessness, and so on.

Pineapple makes you beautiful. In Africa, women use pineapple to fight wrinkles. Pineapple pulp is pureed and applied to the skin as a mask. This removes dead skin cells and allows the cells to renew themselves.

Because of its enzyme bromelain, the pineapple also helps the body burn fat and purify and drain it. It stimulates digestion and helps burn fat very efficiently. That is why it is a top fruit if you want to lose weight.

C3.9.7 Papaya, the all-rounder

In Cameroon, my birthplace, papaya is not only liked as a delicious, low-calorie fruit, but also used as a medicine. International scientific studies support these findings and this knowledge from Africa about the effect of papaya for the health of humans and animals.

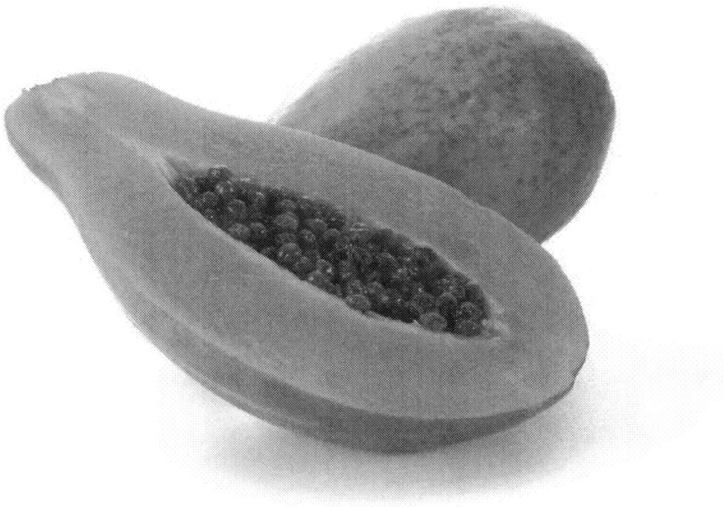

You can use everything on the papaya, the skin of the fruit, the pulp, the black seeds, the leaves and the juice of the tree.

Because of its enzyme papain and the essential nutrients it contains (magnesium, calcium, potassium, manganese, iron, selenium, phosphorus, copper, zinc, fiber), papaya can help against many diseases.

Gastrointestinal complaints, flatulence, constipation, stomach ulcers and parasites and pancreas-related digestive problems are alleviated. The protein-splitting enzyme papain and dietary fiber are responsible for this. The seeds of the papaya are used in Cameroon as an anthelmintic agent.

Papaya helps with:

- Cellulite
- Wrinkles and skin problems
- Wound healing
- Burns
- Unhealthy sperm
- Inflammation, edema and swelling (papaya leaves)
- Rheumatism
- Cancer cells, because of the antioxidants they contain (vitamins, minerals, trace elements, enzymes), which are known to protect our cells by protecting us from free radicals
- And much more

The papaya seeds are even more valuable than the fruit itself. They are also used as a contraceptive in Africa and are very important for the health of certain internal organs, such as the liver.

Isolated chymopapain is used for injection treatment of disc damage.

C3.9.8 Avocado against the cholesterol and leukemia

Avocado is a fruit with very healthy vegetable fat, which contains very important vitamins (A, E, beta and alpha-carotene, biotin). The avocado noticeably improves the absorption of fat-soluble nutrients.

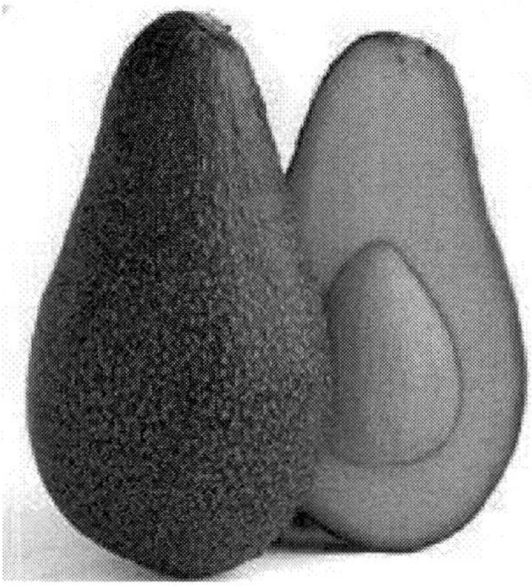

Contrary to the earlier assumption in Western countries that avocado also makes you fat because of its high fat content, many studies, such as the one published in the *Journal of the American Heart Association,* clearly show that avocado does not make you fat, but even lowers cholesterol levels. It is said that just one avocado a day is enough to have a positive effect on cholesterol levels, what also confirms the knowledge of the people in Cameroon. In Cameroon, an avocado is even prepared with vegetable oil so that its vitalizing substances act even faster and stronger in the body. The people in Cameroon are predominantly athletic and muscular.

Avocados may help fight a rare but deadly type of leukemia disease, myeloid leukemia (AML), a study from Canada confirmed. "The fat molecules in avocado attack the stem cells of the leukemia disease, and we must honestly admit that there are few drugs capable of doing this, even today," the researchers said.

Avocado is also used to relieve gastrointestinal discomfort, strengthen teeth and bones and it plays a role in vision and muscle building, my teacher told me during my ritual teaching.

Avocado seeds are also a remedy. I will report in detail about this and other fruits in the forthcoming books "The Healing Power of Tropical Fruits" and "The Healing Power of Foods from the Tropics: Vegetables, Tubers, Herbs, Nuts".

BEWARE: Cultivated tropical fruits no longer have the same effectiveness for health. Avocados from southern Spain, for example, like many tropical fruits from there, are low in vital nutrients. Organic fruits guarantee the most positive results.

C3.9.9 The safou - the unknown wealth of African cuisine

Safou, also called African plum or butter fruit, is the fruit of the safou tree or butter tree, which is native only to Africa, especially Central Africa. The scientific name is Dacryodes edulis. When the fruit is not ripe, it looks pink to slightly reddish. When ripe and ready to eat, it is dark blue. When ripe, it can be eaten raw, boiled in water, or fried. The cooked pulp has a texture similar to butter. The flesh of the fruit contains 48% oil. Safou is a rich source of amino acids and triglycerides and contains various fatty acids: palmitic acid, oleic acid, stearic acid, linolenic acid and linoleic cid.

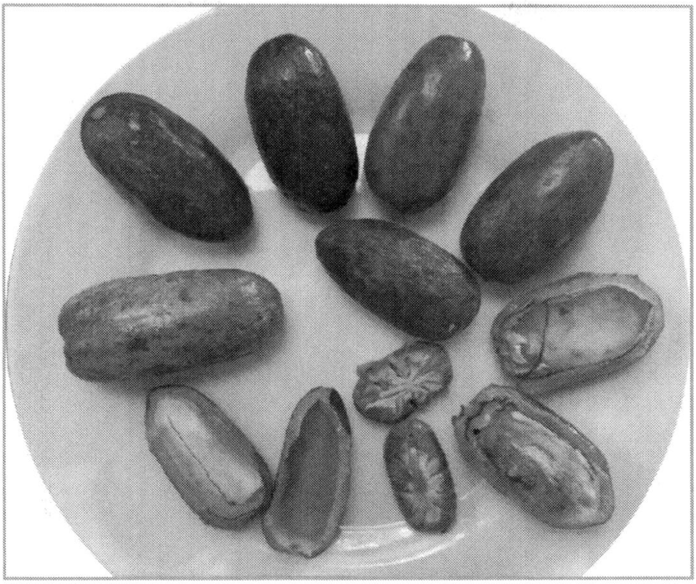

The safou is also rich in vitamins: provitamin A, vitamin E, vitamin C and equally rich in minerals: phosphorus, calcium, manganese, iron, copper, zinc. It is a powerful antioxidant, antibacterial and has several preventive and therapeutic effects: It fights constipation, cancer, osteoporosis, blood lipids, cardiovascular diseases, wounds, intestinal disorders, skin diseases, fever and anxiety.

C3.9.10 Prickly custard apple (Annona muricata): Against cancer par excellence? Better than chemotherapy?

The prickly custard apple, called soursop, is not only considered a delicious fruit in Cameroon, but it is also medicine. When ripe, it is soft and the pulp is snow-white and floury, like butter. It is very rich in vitamins: vitamin C, vitamin B1, B2, B6.

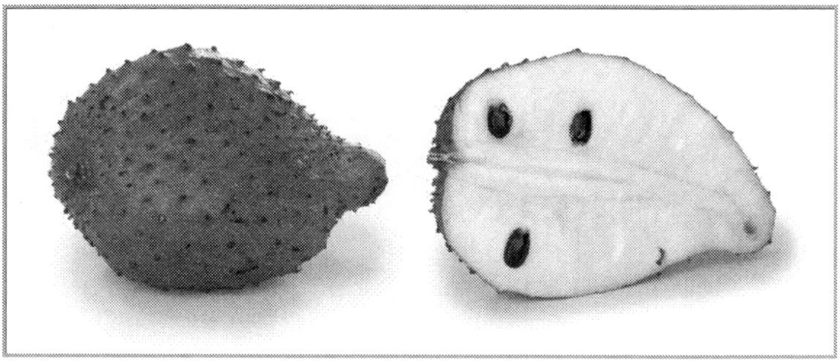

Some naturopaths in Cameroon call this fruit a miracle weapon against cancer. This fruit is said to eliminate cancer cells and, unlike chemotherapy, without attacking healthy cells. Not only the fruit, but the tree itself is said to fight colon, breast, prostate and pancreatic cancer. In Cameroon, the fruit, seeds, leaves, trunk and bark of the fruit are successfully used in natural medicine cancer treatment.

Many of the research results published since the seventies confirm the effect of the fruit against cancer. In 2011, a laboratory test proved that this fruit can successfully inhibit the growth of breast cancer cells. Laboratory research studies published in 2012 showed similar results in pancreatic cancer cells, as Wikipedia writes.

Studies from Asia say that the soursop can eliminate cancer cells up to 10,000 times more effectively than chemotherapy.

The soursop is antimicrobial. This fruit is used in Africa to fight deadly viral, bacterial and fungal infections, parasites and worms. Also, it is among the mixtures that healers give to people who are sick with dengue fever or Ebola. In addition, consuming soursop lowers blood pressure and is a good remedy for depression and stress.

C3.9.11 Citrus fruits: lemons, oranges, grapefruit

Studies have demonstrated an association between citrus fruit consumption and a reduced risk of developing certain cancers, particularly of the esophagus, mouth, larynx and pharynx, intestines, or respiratory organs.

Citrus fruits contain significant amounts of certain polyphenols, flavanoids and a lot of vitamin C (100g of orange contains 50mg of vitamin C and the daily requirement of vitamin C is 80 mg); also many minerals such as iron or phosphorus. They strengthen the immune system and the body's defenses, have an antioxidant and anti-inflammatory effect that can fight cancer and slow down the growth of metastases.

The skin and the white parts of the peel of citrus fruits contain the most flavonoids and limonoids. Grated, you can eat the skin with it, but beware of conventional citrus fruits: Their peels are treated with many chemicals, so it is strongly recommended not to eat this skin along, even if it is washed.

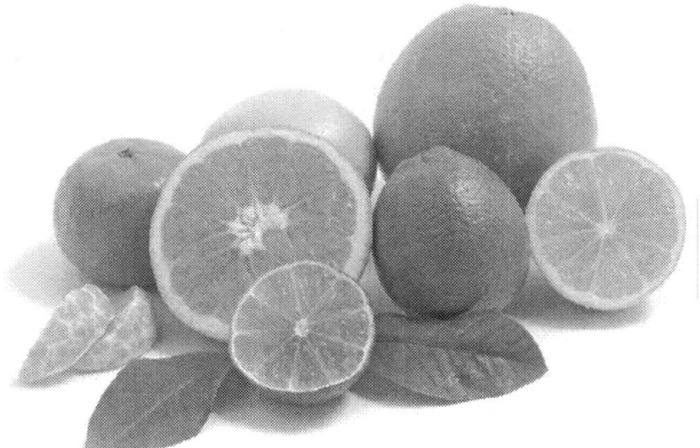

A European study found that a daily intake of 100 ml of citrus juice can reduce throat cancer by 58%, cancer of the mouth and throat by 53%, stomach cancer by 31%, and colon cancer by 18%.

Drinking citrus juices regularly lowers the risk of breast cancer, according to several studies.

Grapefruit is also said to increase the effectiveness of some cancer drugs.

Not all citrus fruits have the same content of healing nutrients. Citrus fruits from greenhouses, which have not had direct contact with the sun, are also not very valuable, because the sun plays a big role in the properties of citrus fruits.

C3.9.12 Uncultivated African mango and wild mango

Mango fruit from the rainforest of West Africa.

The African mango is grown almost exclusively in Africa. A miracle of nature for health. It is a fruit of the mango tree from the rainforest. It differs from the thick, cultivated mango that you can often buy in regular stores by its delicious taste and slender body. The African mangoes have a thin kernel, which is also processed.

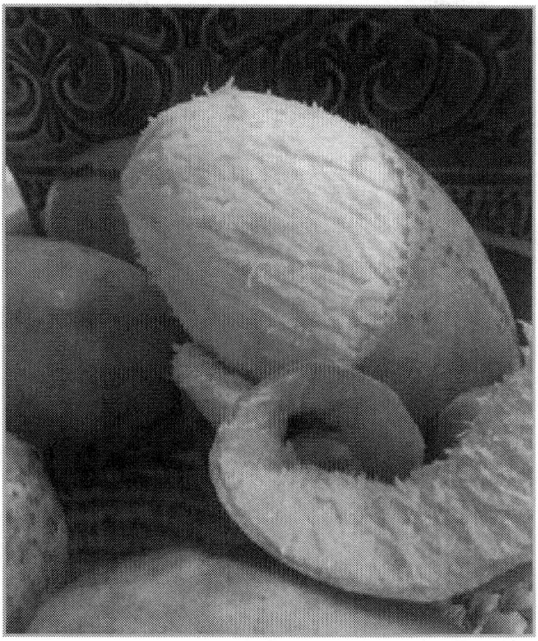

They are a source of many vitamins and other valuable substances:

- Vitamins C and E
- Several B vitamins
- Vitamin K
- Polyphenols
- Provitamin A
- Carotenoids, potassium
- Copper
- 17 amino acids
- 3 and omega 6 polyunsaturated fatty acids

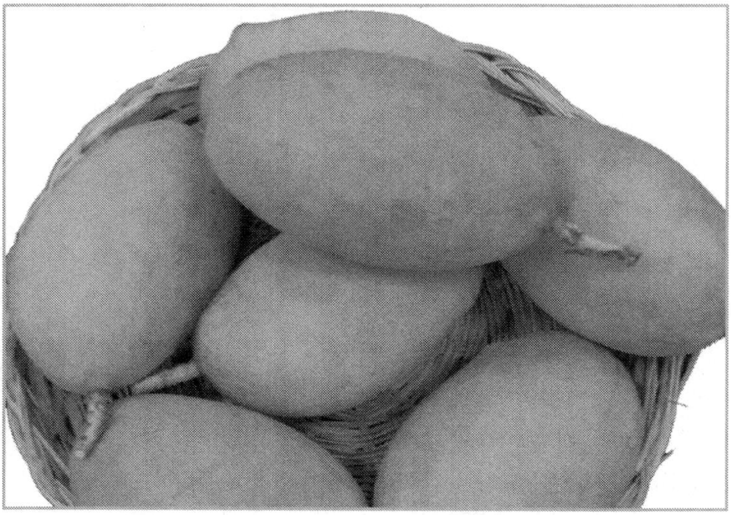

Mango anti-cancer

Tea from mango leaves and mango tree bark, or from crushed kernel are very effective remedies, which I also drank as a child to rid the body of viruses. Harmful toxins are removed from the body and free radicals are kept in check.

The African mango is very rich in polyphenols. These enzymes have antioxidant effects and are involved in the prevention and treatment of cancer, inflammatory diseases, diabetes, cardiovascular or neurodegenerative diseases. It is known that a diet rich in fiber reduces the risk of proliferation of cancer cells in the gastrointestinal tract. African mango is a powerful antioxidant and useful for protecting cells from free radicals. Thus, it reduces the risk of cancer growth.

In addition, studies have shown that lupeol, an enzyme found in African mangoes, directly affects the growth of cancer cells of the prostate and pancreas.

Mango and weight loss

The African mango also fights obesity and thus indirectly cancer. It stimulates the metabolism and effectively burns the fat in the body, thus it optimally supports people in losing weight and weight loss. Due to the high content of vitamin B in the fruit, carbohydrates are transported and broken down faster before they can ruin the figure, according to the literature. The mango contains leptin, which satisfies hunger. The seeds of this fruit are partly responsible for losing weight quickly and healthily. You can grind them and also cook them as a sauce.

MIRACULOUS EFFECT OF POLYPHENOLS CONTAINED IN THE AFRICAN MANGO

Polyphenols are versatile plant compounds (flavones, catechins, tannins) that can treat many diseases. The mixture of polyphenols, vitamins and minerals in African mango effectively release cell receptors, increasing our sensitivity to leptin and insulin and protecting us from producing new fat cells. Polyphenols are also responsible for increasing leptin (a hormone released into the blood where it regulates food intake), despite taking a lower dose of carbohydrates. In addition, the properties of polyphenols intensify the processes of lipolysis. This means that the body uses the accumulated fat reserves to prevent building new ones.

Quote from http://nutrinaafricanmango.de/vorteile-von-african-mango.html

C.3.9.13 Bitacola nut / cola nut

The name bitacola comes from the English *bitter cola*. This nut is bitter and comes from Central Africa. The cola nut is the fruit of the cola tree, which is found in West and Central Africa.

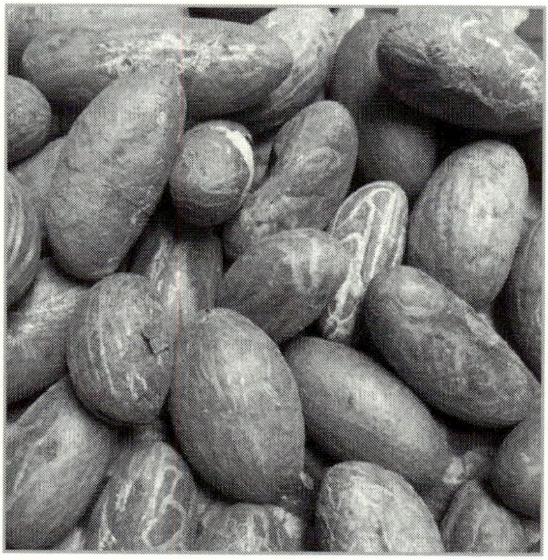

Called "African impotence treatment for man and woman", bitacola is a very effective aphrodisiac, rarely found in nature. It not only increases potency, it inhibits premature ejaculation and you can enjoy your intimate play for hours without "failing". When chewed, the nut is slightly bitter at the beginning, but slightly sweet at the end. However, the bitacola is more than just a sexual enhancer. It is a medicine and strongly alkaline.

The bitacola is eaten in Cameroon every day and quite openly especially by men and in natural medicine, it plays a very important role.

The main active ingredients of cola nuts are caffeine (a caffeine content up to 3.5% higher than coffee) and theobromine. Cola nut extracts are in many cola-containing beverages. However, Coca-Cola has replaced them with cheaper caffeine from coffee.

The cola nut also contains minerals, proteins, sugars, catechin, epicatechin, procyanidins, tannins and starch.

Because of the high caffeine content, the cola nut has a stimulating effect. The caffeine has a different effect than in coffee because it is bound to tannins in the cola nut. Also, the contained "kolatine" and "kolateine" alleviate the effect of caffeine. There is no negative side effect as with coffee (palpitations, insomnia, nervousness, etc.). On the contrary, one feels more calmness, serenity, satisfaction after eating cola nut. You don't feel like eating sweets, you are not hungry and you eat less in general. To conclude, cola nut helps a lot in losing weight.

Cola nut stimulates digestion, lowers high blood pressure and cholesterol, is analgesic, anti-inflammatory, helps with toothache, against migraine, fever, depression and other mental illnesses, is used for its antioxidant effect to fight cancer and other chronic diseases.

You can chew and eat cola nut fresh or mix it into drinks or food as a powder (available on the internet).

C3.9.14 Guava

The guava is a fruit from the guava tree. The skin of the fruit is green but can also be slightly yellowish when too ripe. The pulp is white, yellow or pink with small seeds, depending on the variety.

Everything of the guava (tree, bark, leaves, fruit) is used as a remedy in Cameroon. We drink the tea from leaves and bark to clean the intestinal flora and to get out or kill all harmful little animals and worms. It helps with diarrhea, with toothache and also anesthetizes and disinfects.

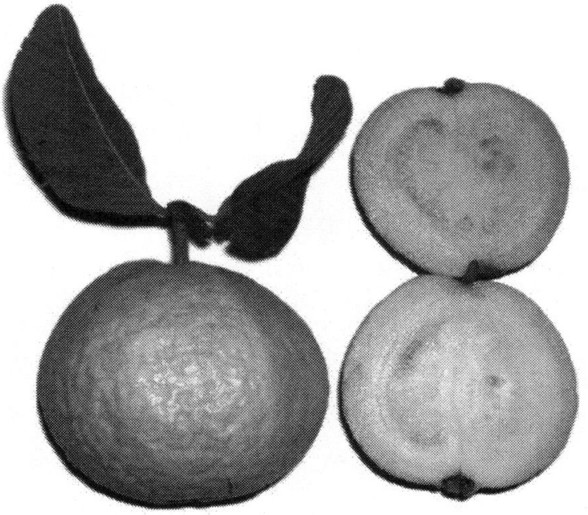

The antioxidant, hepatoprotective (liver-protective), anti-allergenic and antibiotic effects of the leaves, bark and fruit have been scientifically proven and may explain why this fruit is used in Cameroon against inflammation and chronic diseases such as AIDS, Ebola and cancer.

Natural medicine practitioners dry the fruit and leaves and make a powder from them, which they give to people suffering from serious diseases.

Guava juice can be bought everywhere and it is highly recommended. The fruit contains calcium, iron, vitamin A, vitamin B, vitamin C (more than oranges and citrus fruits) and is rich in pectins. The leaves and bark of the guava tree contain tannins, which have astringent, anti-inflammatory, antibacterial, antiviral effects and neutralize toxins. They also contain essential oil. All this makes the guava a real anti-cancer food.

C3.9.15 Monkey bread, strong remedy for chronic diseases

Monkey bread is the fruit of the baobab, a powerful remedy for chronic diseases. This fruit is secretly in many medicines that people have to take today to fight or cure diseases like cancer, Alzheimer's disease, diabetes, etc. Many athletes feed on this fruit with amazing healing properties.

The fruit is the source of many micronutrients and antioxidants. It contains vitamins A, C, B1, B2, B6, PP, minerals, such as calcium (twice as much as milk), phosphorus, iron, potassium, zinc, amino acids, such as proline and L-histidine, more than 13 essential amino acids and has always been used in Africa against chronic diseases.

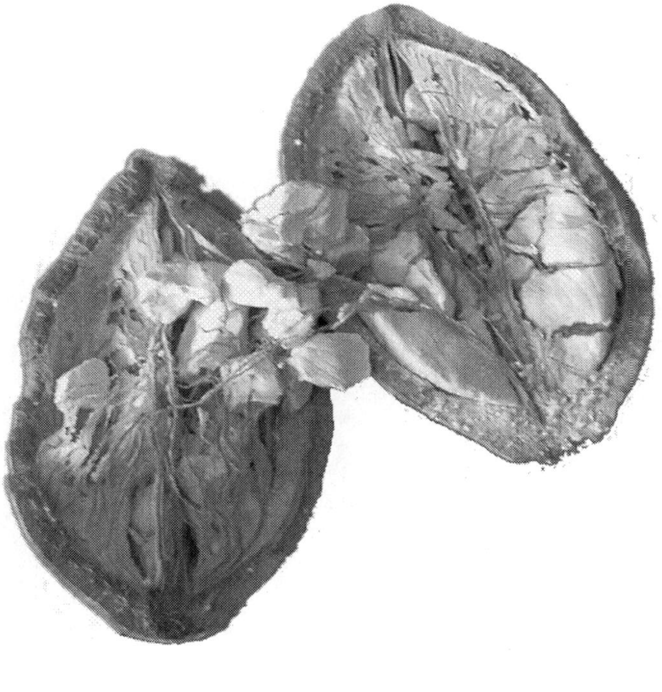

Due to its balanced content of hydrophilic (vitamin C, flavonoids) and lipophilic antioxidants (beta-carotene), the flesh of the baobab tree is a truly global and effective antioxidant. It protects all cell structures from free radicals and successfully fights the development and spread of cancer.

C3.9.16 Hot chili peppers, a powerful anti-cancer vegetable and one of the best medicines around

Spicy food attacks sharp. Two varieties of chilies that are much used and applied as strong medicine in Africa are the Habaneros in different species and the African Bird's Eye chilies.

My natural medicine practitioner in Cameroon rated the spicy plants as excellent remedies for many chronic diseases. He praised African hot chilies and said that Europeans would be much better off, health-wise, if they only ate spicy foods. Their bodies would ward off many chronic diseases on their own. The spicy and healing effect of chili peppers has to do with the active ingredient capsaicin they contain.

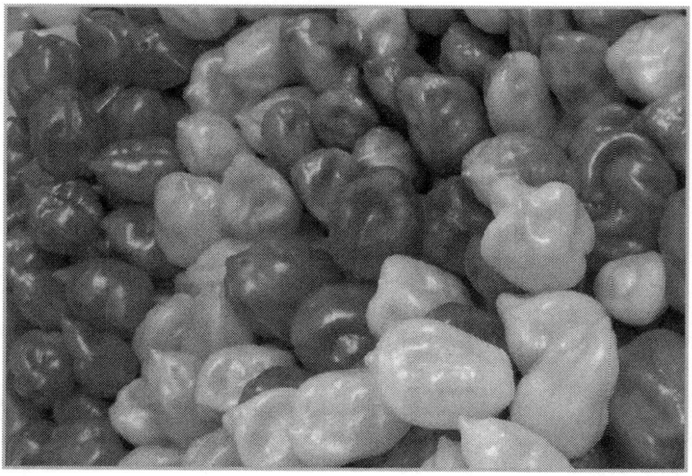

Hot chili peppers against cancer

So this medical doctor in Cameroon used chili to fight cancer or to stop its spread. Especially men with prostate complaints and prostate cancer were regular customers of his chili therapy.

Scientific studies go in the same direction and prove that fresh chili peppers have an anti-cancer effect. They inhibited the growth of cancer cells and would protect the cells from cancer. They activate the suicide program of cancer cells, called apoptosis, and thus the diseased cells no longer grow, they simply die out. Metastases are thus also prevented.

A study, published in December 2008 by researchers at the University of Pittsburgh School of Medicine, proves that capsaicin is also an agent against pancreatic cancer. They found that capsaicin programs cancer cells to eventually kill them.

Hot peppers also help fight breast cancer, as researchers from Changhua Christian Hospital in Changhua, Taiwan reported in an October 2011 study. As www.zentrum-der-gesundheit.de/capsaicin-ia.html writes, here too, the hot chilies attack cancer cells in a similar way as they do pancreatic cancer:

When breast cancer suddenly stops responding to chemotherapy or radiation, this is often a sign of a malfunctioning caspase-3. Caspase-3 is an enzyme that - together with other enzymes - recognizes when a cell is very sick, very old or even irreparably damaged. Caspase-3 organizes the death of this cell in such a case.

If caspase-3 remains inactive, the cells no longer die - no matter how sick or how damaged they are. In cancer cells, caspase-3 is no longer active. Therefore, they can proliferate and eventually form tumors and metastases.

Capsaicin breaks this cycle. It prevents cell growth even in those cells that no longer have caspase-3 and triggers their suicide program.

In addition, habaneros contain significant amounts of vitamin C and vitamin A, both of which have antioxidant effects that can reduce the risk of cancer by inhibiting the DNA-damaging effects of free radicals. Even a small piece of pepper in food is enough to reach the daily dose of vitamin C.

Here are more healthy properties of chili peppers:

- They are rich in vitamins C and A and are excellent antioxidants and tough opponents of free radicals. Thus, they protect the body from harm. The hotter the natural plant, the healthier it is. But still, you should not overdose them when eating.
- They regulate blood sugar.
- They are sexual teasers. They strengthen the potency and libido.
- They stimulate the metabolism, melt body fat and thus help in weight loss.
- They lower the cholesterol level.
- They are anti-inflammatory.
- They thin the blood.
- They protect the stomach and gastric mucosa.
- They are also used in Africa to combat depression.
- They protect the liver.

Not everything that is hot helps. Fresh chilies are particularly suitable. Paprika powder - especially if it is not organic - helps less and can even be carcinogenic because of the toxins it contains (pesticides).

C3.9.17 Pumpkin and pumpkin seeds from Africa against prostate cancer

Pumpkin seeds from Africa are full of healthy ingredients. Cameroonian pumpkin seeds are white and come from edible pumpkins. They are real remedies, even against chronic inflammation and infection.

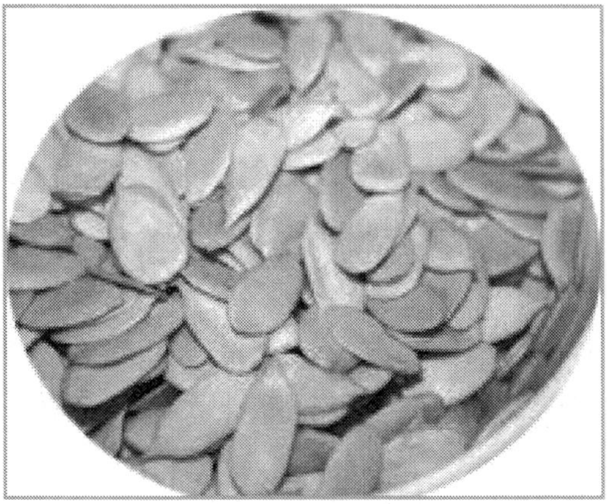

They contain many vitamins (A, B1, B2, B5, C, D, E), many minerals (copper, manganese, phosphorus, zinc, iron, potassium, magnesium) and a lot of fiber.

Epidemiological studies show an association between pumpkin consumption and a reduced risk of certain types of cancer.

Pumpkin seeds contain a large amount of phytosterols. These substances have a very positive effect on health: against cardiovascular problems and prostate enlargement. They are used in Africa for certain preparations against many types of cancer and especially prostate and breast cancer.

Pumpkin seeds contain many antioxidants, such as carotenoids (beta-carotene, lutein and zeaxanthin, beta-cryptoxanthin), the consumption of which is believed to be associated with a lower risk of cancer.

In addition, pumpkin and pumpkin seeds lower blood sugar and act against cystitis and diabetes.

The oil of pumpkin seeds is also very valuable.

C3.9.18 African carbohydrates: the most effective anti-cancer foods

I will mainly mention food that you can buy everywhere in Asian and Afro stores and also in well-stocked food markets.

You will quickly understand with the properties of these foods why few people in Africa suffer from so-called diet-related cancer. These foods are not those that are eaten only by chance and by the way, like fruit in Western countries, they rather are part of daily use: morning, noon, night, in between. This means that people provide their bodies with anti-cancer foods all day long and thus protect themselves from cancer or thus push back cancer and slow down or stop its spread.

It is no coincidence that the pharmaceutical industry uses many of these foods in its drugs, even if it does not always declare this clearly. Of course, it wants its drugs to be sold. Cancer therapy combined with these foods and the teachings of natural medicine can help the sick very much, because all these foods do not interfere with drug therapy in any case but can significantly slow down the spread of cancer.

Almost without exception, all these staple foods from Africa contain nitrilosides or vitamin B17.

Roots and tubers

- **Yam**

Contains the famous vitamin B17, which according to some studies, kills cancer cells in humans.

The yam is a large root of the yam plant. Its skin is brown and the inside is yellow or white. It grows in tropical countries. The root is peeled and eaten boiled or fried in different variations and forms as a garnish to different sauces.

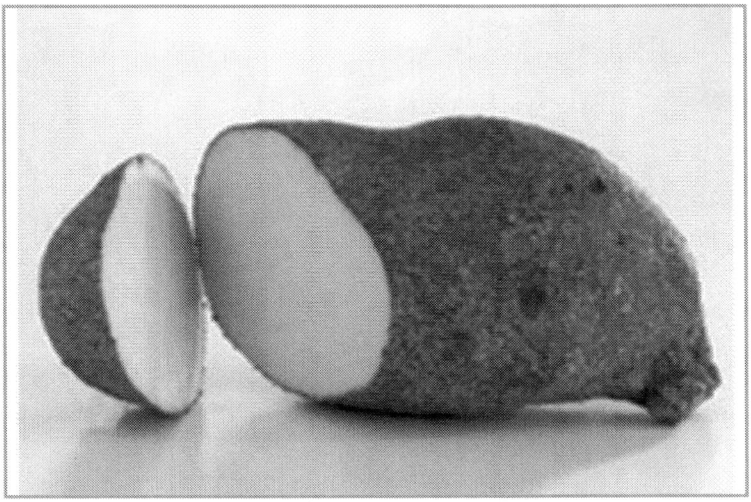

Yam is used as a remedy in Cameroon. Its sticky liquid is extracted too, to cure chronic diseases. Yam root, yam leaves and stems are anti-cancer agents in natural medicine. Yam also helps against osteoporosis, thrombosis, diabetes, mental illnesses such as depression, stress and much more, as well as to lose weight. When I was a child and had muscle pain, my mother massaged me with yam and a few minutes later all the pain was gone.

Yam is low in fat, quite rich in vitamin C and contains other important substances: alkaloids, tannins, sapogenins such as diosgenin, which the pharmaceutical industry likes to use.

Scientific studies on animals may confirm why Africans use yam as a remedy. Experiments on animals with diosgenin showed amazing results. Diosgenin is an antioxidant that effects the inflammatory system, against microbes and viruses, against cancer (in animal studies it has been found to inhibit cell growth of colon and breast cancer cells) and lowers cholesterol levels.

Yam also acts against joint inflammation, rheumatic inflammation and against osteoporosis.

Yam increases libido and is very effective in helping women with menopausal symptoms.

The leaves of yam tree are a delicious vegetable with many vitamins and minerals.

- **Cassava (manioc)**

Cassava also contains the vitamin B17.

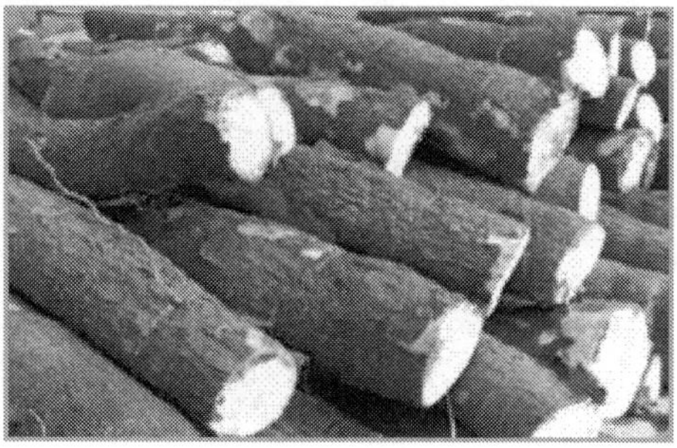

Report of a cancer patient who was cured with cassava:

This letter is about how manioc, which also contains Vitamin B17, has the potential to combat cancer.
My story starts with a cancer I developed seven years ago. A cystoscopy revealed transitional cell cancer. The kidney, ureter and a little part of the bladder where the ureter enters the bladder were surgically removed. I was given radiation treatment, and I remained in good health over the next seven years (I was examined once a year). My bladder was cancer-free until November 2009. That month I started passing blood. Another cystoscopy was done, and a polypoidal growth close to the bladder neck was removed. The biopsy this time again revealed transitional cell cancer.

I had read on world without cancer.org that manioc - also known as cassava or tapioca - has a high B17 component. For a whole month following the removal of the polypoidal growth in the bladder, I ate manioc daily, usually twice a day. A cystoscopy done a month later showed that the bladder was completely symptom-free. I felt very well.

Was my wellbeing the result of the cancer-fighting properties of manioc's Vitamin B17? It would be wonderful, I thought, if a test group of cancer patients used manioc in order to confirm that manioc really does have the ability to fight cancer, as it seemed to have done in my case.

Here is what happens when a cancer patient eats manioc:

Once the manioc is consumed, the manioc's Vitamin B17 combines in the normal human cell with an enzyme called Rhodanese, which breaks down the B17 into three sugars. The cancer cell, which is an immature cell, has a different enzyme, beta-glucosidase, which breaks the B17 into glucose, benzaldehyde and hydrocyanic acid. The hydrocyanic acid acts like an LTTE cyanide capsule, killing the cancer cell.

I appeal to all cancer patients to try the manioc solution. If it works, it could be a great discovery for cancer patients around the world, especially those living in the tropics of Asia, Africa and the Americas, where manioc / cassava / tapioca grows and is freely available. Dr. Cynthia Jayasuriya, Ear, Nose and Throat Surgeon

***http://www.sundaytimes.lk/100207/Plus/plus_03.html

Cassava, like yam, is a root that is very popular in Africa, especially in Central Africa and Cameroon. It is, like all roots, a very important food in Africa, eaten almost daily in various forms. The leaves are prepared in Cameroon as a delicious vegetable.

In various reports, one can read that cassava is toxic in its raw state because of the cyanogenic glycoside it contains. This is not entirely true. It depends on which cassava you eat. We sometimes eat cassava raw, but you can't eat much of it at all. The problem is solved naturally because it just doesn't taste good raw. Raw cassava is a bit like potato. For the poison to work you would have to eat way too much of it. But this substance, labeled poison, is at the same time considered a strong remedy in Cameroon's natural medicine, especially for chronic inflammations like cancer. In fact, cassava is mainly eaten boiled, fried or dried and has amazing healing properties. The dangerous cassava root is not the one we get to buy everywhere here, but the "wild" cassava variety. This one is really poisonous. You have to be careful! But you would have to go to Brazil to find this one. The risk is therefore very small, almost non-existent.

Cassava and cassava leaves help against burns, conjunctivitis, anemia.

During my research with natural medicine practitioners in Cameroon, I learned that cassava is recommended for chronic inflammation and also as a cancer preventative. They all said that the leaves of cassava would also be a miracle for the body.

Now, when I analyzed scientific studies and the properties of cassava, I found out why this assumption of Cameroonian naturopaths could be true. Cassava contains a large amount of vitamin B17, also vitamins B1, B2, B3, B5, B6, B7, B9, B12 (folic acid), vitamin C, vitamin K, calcium, chlorine, potassium, magnesium, sodium, phosphorus, sulfur, iron fluorine, copper, iodine, manganese, zinc, many amino acids - all substances that cancer is afraid of and that help to protect against this disease or limit its spread and development. The effect of cassava against cancer is also reflected in the fact that cassava contains many antioxidants.

- **Taro**

Taro is considered a staple food in Cameroon, just like yam, plantain and cassava. Taro is the name given to the plant itself, but also to the edible tuber, which is also known as dasheen. In general, taro can be prepared similarly to potatoes. In Cameroon, the tubers are boiled in water and only then peeled. Taro is not edible raw and is very slimy.

The nutritional values of taro alone show how healthy and beneficial it can be:
Vitamins: vitamin A, beta-carotene, vitamin B1, vitamin B2,

vitamin B3, vitamin B5, vitamin B6, vitamin B7, vitamin B9, total folic acid, vitamin C, vitamin K.

Minerals: calcium, chlorine, potassium, magnesium, sodium, phosphorus S, sulfur

Trace elements: iron, fluorine, iodine, copper, manganese, zinc

Taro is an anti-cancer food. Taro root plays a significant role in antioxidant activities in our body. There are many vitamins and various phenolic antioxidants in this root. They strengthen our immune system and help fight dangerous free radicals. Free radicals are created during cell metabolism and they can cause healthy cells to mutate into cancer cells.

Taro is also effective against diabetes, against cataracts, for intestinal problems, cleanses the intestinal flora and much more.

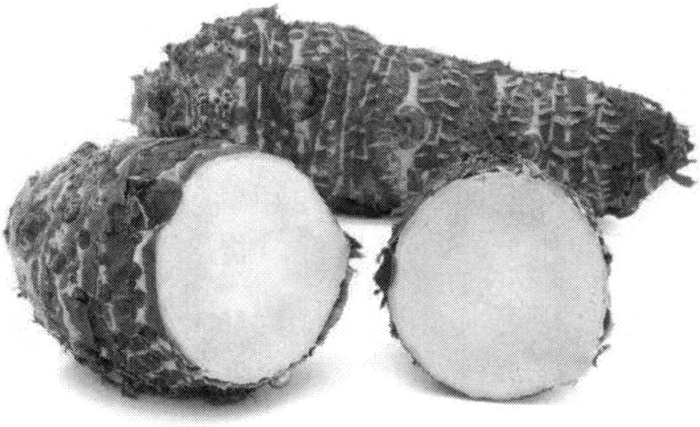

- **Cocoyam, macabo**

Macabo is also a root and is very similar to taro. It is only firmer and less slimy.

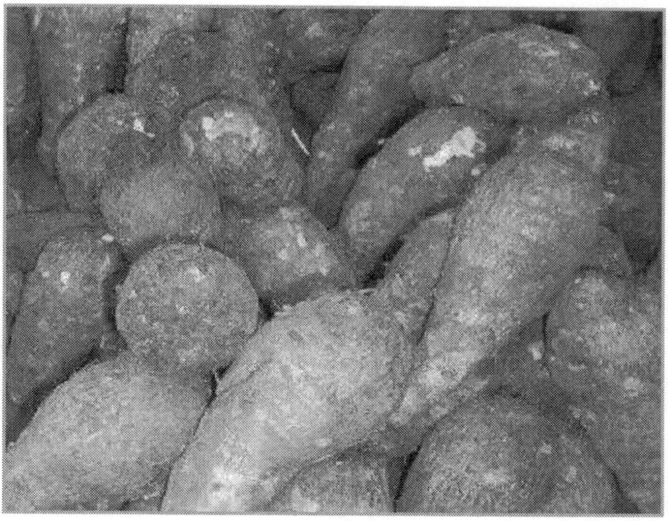

Plantain

Plantain is the fruit of the banana tree, which grows in tropical and subtropical regions.

Plantain is to the people of Africa, in Cameroon, as pasta or white flour is to Westerners. Plantain is eaten every day and several times a day, boiled, fried, roasted, dried. Green, it tastes almost like potato, ripe it is yellow and tastes similar to banana.

Plantain may be just a normal food for many, but it has amazing healing properties due to its amazing properties. Plantain is literally a food medicine.

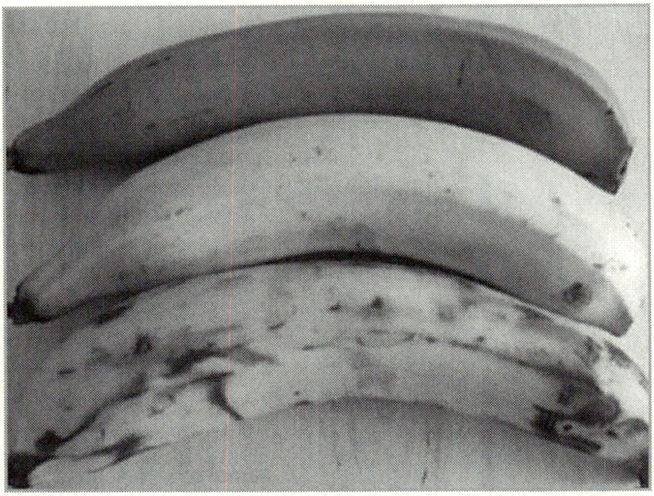

Everything that plantain is:

- It is source of strength and energy
- It is almost fat free
- It is rich in fiber
- It is rich in vitamins: vitamin A, retinol, carotene, vitamin B1, vitamin B2, vitamin B3, vitamin B5, vitamin B6, vitamin B7, vitamin B9 (folic acid), vitamin C, vitamin E, vitamin K.
- It is rich in minerals: Calcium, chlorine, potassium, magnesium, sodium, phosphorus, sulfur.
- It is rich in trace elements: Iron, fluorine, iodine, copper, manganese, zinc
- It is rich in amino acids
- It is rich in antioxidants
- It is alkaline
- It contains resistant starch

Everything plantain can do:

Plantain acts against:

- Kidney and bladder problems
- Menstrual cramps
- Osteoporosis
- Heart disease
- Anemia
- Nerve inflammation
- Free radicals

And it heals the intestine and frees it from bacterial pathogens!

C4. SEX and exercise: Not food, but as natural remedies they also help against mental and physical diseases

Exercise is a good support for losing weight.

Sports and exercise help to strengthen the muscles and stimulate the metabolism, which leads to accelerate and increase the burning of fat.

I think moderate engaging in sport activity is best, firstly so that you don't lose the motivation again very quickly and secondly because you immediately gain weight again if you first do a lot of exercise and then no more.

Especially if you already were fat, it is advisable to combine losing weight with exercising, so that afterwards you do not look thin, but for that the skin hangs.

For exercise, it's enough to jog a little, walk a little, go for a walk more often, and get things done by foot (don't drive somewhere you can also walk to). Get a trampoline and use it at home every time you have a few minutes: You'll be amazed at how a little exercise does your body and soul good.

Sex alone, in my opinion, does not help that much with weight loss. But certain sex practices do. If sex is active and intense, with lots of movements and changing positions, and lasts at least 10 minutes, it can also cause calories to be burned.

C5 Toxins in food, countermeasures and alternatives

http://www.gesundheitstabelle.de/index.php/schadstoffe-gifte/gifte-lebensmittel

Poison	Recommendations what to do	Alternatives
Acrylamide	Infrequent consumption of potato chips, do not heat French fries / fried food above 175°C. French fries preferably light, thick, juicy, than thin, dark and dry.	E.g. corn chips instead of potato chips
Agaritine	Do not eat raw mushrooms! Agaritine is destroyed during cooking/frying (from 70°C).	Cooked mushrooms. Do not eat uncooked, dried mushrooms
Alcohol (ethanol)	Do not drink every day, never "get drunk" if possible	THC; have fun without drugs ;)
Anthraquinone	Drink black and green tea less often for the time being, wait until problem is solved....	Other teas, mainly organic teas (organic black tea, however, does not contain less anthraquinone)
Antibiotics	Eat little or no meat. Reduce consumption of dairy products. Seafood from aquaculture, organic only	Meat and dairy products from organic production (organic animals may only receive antibiotics once in their lifetime)

Poison	Recommendations what to do	Alternatives
Aluminum	Avoid acidic foods in particular that come into contact with aluminum.	Steel cooking pots, drinks in glass bottles instead of cans
Arsenic	Wash or soak rice before cooking and strain off the water! Particularly contaminated: Rice from Asia	Husked rice less loaded, parboiled rice higher, whole grain rice highest.
Aspartame	Consumption of aspartame should be avoided: suspected of causing cancer. Questionable for allergy sufferers. Many different opinions and assessments!	Instead, sugar in moderation or stevia
Azo dyes	Colored foods and candies that are bright red or yellow are often colored with azo dyes	Natural food colors
BHT	Avoid frequent intake.	Products without BHT
Benzene	Avoid foods that contain both benzoic acid as a preservative and ascorbic acid!	Products without benzoic acid.

Poison	Recommendations what to do	Alternatives
Benzoic acid Sodium benzoate	Reduce consumption, especially if E 210 is contained in beverages with ascorbic acid. E number: E 211	Preservatives usually not absolutely necessary
Bisphenol A (BPA)	Dissolves from plastic when heated in microwave or kettle!	Polyethylene packaging usually does not contain BPA. Incidentally, the substitute BPS is just as harmful.
Cadmium	Organic foods have lower levels of cadmium because cadmium attaches to phosphate (artificial fertilizer). Dark chocolate from South America much more contaminated than African. Eat less chocolate.	Organic food, African chocolate (attention: child labor)
Cholesterol		None. Cholesterol is an important substance. Tip: Do not consume meat, or greatly reduce animal fats in the diet.

Poison	Recommendations what to do	Alternatives
Coumarin	Avoid products with cassia cinnamon. Official limit for coumarin: no more than 4 cinnamon cookies for children per day!	Ceylon cinnamon, other spices
Cyclamate	Avoid cyclamate.	Sugar in moderation, stevia
Fungicides	Be careful with Caipirhina with non-bio limes! Wash fruits, vegetables well!	
Hardened fats	Avoid margarine and convenience foods.	Olive oil, organic margarine without hydrogenated fats, butter
Genetically modified food	Avoid genetically modified foods and fight them politically.	Conventional, cross-bred foodstuffs
Saturated fatty acids		Vegetable fats, especially thistle, olive, rapeseed and sunflower oil. Reduce the consumption of animal fats!

Poison	Recommendations what to do	Alternatives
Glutamate / flavor enhancers		High-quality food does not need any flavor enhancers. Yeast extract contains less glutamate than the industrially produced E-621.
Glycidamide	Infrequent consumption of potato chips, do not heat French fries / fried food above 175°C. French fries prefer light, thick, juicy, rather than thin, dark and dry. Frying oil should contain little unsaturated fatty acids.	E.g. corn chips instead of potato chips
Glyphosate	Glyphosate is a suspected carcinogen and is a critical health risk through daily human ingestion.	Organic food! For the production of food from conventional agriculture, pesticides containing glyphosate are very often used.
Histamine		Avoid these foods, reduce consumption. Especially red wine. Histamine-free wine is available for purchase.

Poison	**Recommendations what to do**	**Alternatives**
Melamine		Melamine dishes can be used well without heating. Alternatives, of course, porcelain and earthenware.
Methanol		Drink less alcohol, or prefer less loaded drinks to higher loaded ones.
Mineral oil (MOSH / MOAH)		Do not eat food that has had direct contact with printed or recycled paper packaging.
Sodium nitrite, nitrite curing salt	Never heat sausage/cheese with nitrite above 130 degrees! Never cover pizza with salami, ham or Gouda! Otherwise carcinogenic nitrosamines are produced during digestion. Dangerous for babies.	Cheese and sausage with other preservatives or unpreserved
Sodium fluoride, fluorine	Avoid all products with fluorides!!!	Sea salt (and toothpaste) without additives

Poison	Recommendations what to do	Alternatives
Natamycin	Do not eat cheese rind under any circumstances, unless it is explicitly designated as edible on the packaging. Separate the rind and 5 mm from the cheese and throw away, as natamycin also diffuses into the cheese.	Organic cheese does not contain natamycin.
Nitrate		Prefer less affected vegetables. Especially in the winter months.
Patent blue		-
PET bottles: Acetaldehyde / Estrogen		Glass bottles! PET bottles are superfluous.
Phthalates	Always avoid packages with plasticizers! Above all, eat not much canned food.	Plastics without plasticizers, alternative packaging materials

Poison	Recommendations what to do	Alternatives
Phytoestrogens	Do not eat too much soy and not every day. With normal consumption, the positive health properties clearly outweigh the benefits. Children should eat only a **little** soy products.	For vegetarians: Instead of tofu also eat an egg, cheese, seitan, falafel from time to time.
Polycyclic hydrocarbons (PAH)	Avoid grilled foods. Especially the black parts! Reduce consumption of smoked foods.	Roast instead of grill. Gas grill instead of coal grill, prefer unsmoked food.
Pyrrolizidine alkaloids	Avoid foods in the production of which toxic plants can be mixed with the food plants (unfortunately, this is also very often the case with herbal teas).	Food where you can be sure about the origin. Organic teas are rarely contaminated with this substance.
Radioactivity	Avoid appropriate foods and continue to inform yourself about how radiation levels develop, e.g. in Pacific fish (pollock / fish sticks!).	Food from other regions / fishing areas (fish).

Poison	Recommendations what to do	Alternatives
Saccharin		Instead, sugar in moderation or stevia.
Safrole		Avoid these foods or consume only in small amounts.
Mold toxin / Aflatoxins etc.	Throw away moldy food! Especially those from cereals, vegetables, fruits (in cheese you can generously cut it off).	Buy susceptible food from trustworthy countries (keyword: good storage)
Melting salts, phosphates	Do not eat. Omit for hamburgers	Good cheese does not contain melting salts and tastes much better.
Semicarbazid e		Coatings without plasticizers (e.g. polyethylene, polypropylene. Foodstuffs without appropriate packaging.
Silicones		Pure vegetable frying oil without additives

Poison	Recommendations what to do	Alternatives
Solanine	Cut out stems of tomato and do not eat. Generously cut off any sprouts from potatoes. Do not eat green potatoes or tomatoes!	
Stevia		Little sugar
Sulfites		Wine without artificially added sulfites
Trans fatty acids		Avoid high-risk foods
Vanillin		Real vanilla, abandon the aroma
Caramel coloring (ammonium sulfite)	There are no limits, but should be avoided.	Beverages without colorants or with natural colorants such as malt extract

C6 Tips for vegans and vegetarians

Food | Theme	Occurrence | Use	Tips | Alternatives
Terms 'Vegan' and 'Vegetarian'	Terms are not protected.	Look carefully at what ingredients are listed on products. You should generally inform yourself carefully if you are a vegetarian or vegan.
Beeswax / Honey	Beeswax is used as a coating agent in many sweets. Honey is eaten pure and is found in many finished products and sweets.	Vegans mostly avoid products with honey or beeswax content. Beekeeping is seen as negative by many vegans.
Eggs	Male chicks are usually sorted out and killed directly after hatching. This also applies explicitly to almost all organic eggs!	In some organic stores you can also find eggs from an animal husbandry that leaves male chicks alive (at least until slaughter). The only truly animal-friendly option for egg consumption is eggs from farmyard chickens that are not kept for slaughter and where the roosters are not killed either.
Iron	Consideration should be given to iron in vegetarian and vegan diets.	Those who are vegan should pay at least some attention to eating iron-rich plant foods on a regular basis.

Food | Theme	Occurrence | Use	Tips | Alternatives
Meat substitutes	Vegetarians and vegans usually (just like their carnivorous peers) have a need for the flavor note "umami". As a substitute for meat, vegetable meatballs or tofu, soy meatballs and seitan, which are very similar in terms of consistency, are particularly suitable. However, the preparation is important, otherwise they taste bland.	Tip for tofu/soy meatballs: Season with plenty of soy sauce, cumin and coriander. Then fry in a pan with plenty of oil and finely chopped onions (soak soy cutlets in boiling water beforehand).
Fruit juices and lemonades	Clear fruit juices are usually filtered with gelatin (partly fish gelatin). The gelatin is no longer contained in the end product.	Direct juices, freshly squeezed juices. Lemonades without juice content.

Food | Theme	Occurrence | Use	Tips | Alternatives
Gelatin (E 441)	Wine gum/gummy bears, chewy candies, pudding, etc. Animal: From dead pig or cattle (skin). **Caution:** Also found in many medications, analog film rolls and in photo paper. Also in paintball ammunition.	Pectin, agar-agar, starch, locust bean gum, kelp algae. Some soft candies such as licorice do not contain gelatin.
Glycerin (E 422)	Glycerin is partly of animal origin.	Most glycerin is of vegetable origin. Among other things, it is produced as a residual material in biodiesel production.
Medication	Very many pills and tablets have a shell made of gelatin.	Many drugs are also available with non-animal shells.
Cheese (rennet)	Many cheeses are made with rennet and are therefore NOT VEGETARIAN!	When buying cheese, make sure that the package says "made with microbiological rennet".
Margarine	Attention: Margarines are not always vegetarian or vegan. Sometimes they are enriched with fish oil (omega-3 margarines) or whey.	Observe the list of ingredients on the packaging!

Food | Theme	Occurrence | Use	Tips | Alternatives
Omega-3 fatty acids	Food supplements often made from fish and or seals.	Plant carriers of omega-3 fatty acids are available. E.g. in flaxseed oil, chia oil, perilla oil, etc.
Dairy products	Vegetarians often eat dairy products. Here, a reduction in intake can be useful for health and animal welfare reasons.	There is a suspected link between milk consumption and cancer. Also objectionable: Animal welfare in factory farming.
Proteins / Protein	Proteins are important for a balanced diet. Even for vegetarians and vegans there is actually no deficiency. Nevertheless, one should pay attention to the daily intake of protein-containing plant foods as well.	
Shellac (E 904)	Harmless tree resin taken from the tree by lice. Possibly problematic for vegans. Vegetarians should generally have little sympathy for lice :)	Used as a plastic substitute, furniture care or food supplement. Alternatives are mostly chemical.

Food | Theme	Occurrence | Use	Tips | Alternatives
Sebum	Animal fat that is an ingredient in many cosmetics, bird feed, candles (stearin), lubricants (e.g. for stringed instruments) and, in some cases, vegetarian dishes. Do not confuse with mineral talc in food (E-553b).	Purely plant-based cosmetics. Natural cosmetics usually have no animal ingredients.
Taurine	Taurine is usually found as an additive in energy drinks. According to marketing, it supposedly increases concentration, but this is not scientifically proven. Taurine is a substance that occurs in mammals, but there is also synthetically produced taurine.	For vegetarians and vegans, the taurine in energy drinks is harmless because it is synthetically produced.

Food | Theme	Occurrence | Use	Tips | Alternatives
Animal testing	Animal testing is mostly used in medical/pharmaceutical research. Less frequently also for the development of cosmetics.	For cosmetics, there are lists of companies that do not use animal testing. Animal testing for medicines and basic research can be difficult to prevent from the consumer's point of view.
Vitamin A	Two-thirds of most people's vitamin A intake comes from meat and dairy products. Deficiency is rare.	Vegans should make sure to eat enough plant foods containing the vitamin A precursor carotene (provitamin A).
Vitamin B12	Vegetarians usually cover their vitamin B12 needs through dairy products and eggs.	Anyone who is vegan should be concerned about sufficient vitamin B12 intake. This cannot be guaranteed via purely plant-based food.
Vitamin D and vitamin D3 preparations	Vitamin D3 is always of animal origin. Obtained either from fish, milk, eggs or animal fats.	Synthetic production is also possible.

Food | Theme	Occurrence | Use	Tips | Alternatives
Wine	Animal additives. Cheap wine and most clear juices are filtered with gelatin from dead pigs or fish. Gelatin is no longer present in the final product, but was used in its production.	There are manufacturers who filter the wine differently. This is especially true for more expensive wines or when it is stated on the packaging (Vegan).
Wool / wool grease	Wool usually from sheep. Wool fat partly also contained in cosmetics.	Basically all right. If applicable, questionable animal husbandry. Sheep (like other breeding animals) are also usually slaughtered long before their natural life expectancy.
Additives	Many food additives (E-numbers) contain animal components without the consumer necessarily being aware of this. The most important ones are listed in this table, all others can be taken from corresponding tables.	Those who want to be sure which natural additives are of animal origin should study the relevant tables.

Food | Theme	Occurrence | Use	Tips | Alternatives
Sugar (refined)	Refined sugar is partly decolorized with animal charcoal in some countries (e.g. USA). This is not done in Germany.	Normally, little thought needs to be given to this subject in Germany. In other countries, research whether animal charcoal is commonly used in sugar production.

Source: with support from http://gesundheitstabelle.de/index.php/2012-11-04-20-02-49/tips-fuer-vegetarier-veganer

Insider Tip:

The Africans or the Cameroonians eat very vegetarian and also vegan. In Cameroon, almost all typical vegetarian and vegan dishes are prepared with palm oil. Look for cooking recipes in chapter D9.

D. Nutrition against diet-related cancer

Experts estimate that breast cancer, ovarian cancer, uterine cancer, colon cancer, prostate cancer, stomach cancer, liver cancer and pancreatic cancer are directly related to poor diet. It is said that about 1/3 of all cancer cases could be prevented by a healthier diet.

My evaluation of many studies shows that people who eat a predominantly alkaline diet, with many antioxidant-rich foods, with sufficient essential fatty acids, regularly consumed fruit, healthy meat and fish, have a significantly lower risk of cancer than other people who do not eat these healthy foods. This effect increases the more athletically active people are.

The natural doctors in Cameroon advise that the diet must be holistic and should contain foods from all food groups. The more varied the diet, the more impressive the protection against and the fight against cancer. It doesn't do much good to always alternate between two healthy foods all week, or to eat a fundamentally poor diet and then eat an apple every day. It's also dangerous to think you're eating healthy when you eat a salad. More important is the dressing. The salad dressing you get everywhere is much worse than not eating a salad at all.

D1 Prevention against cancer is in our diet and in our psyche: what to watch out for

The best cancer prevention and support of any cancer therapy is diet and a healthy lifestyle. As I mentioned, not only a toxic-free diet protects us from cancer or fights cancer, but also the choice and type of food.

Diet can prevent cancer. By eating certain foods, you can reduce the risk of cancer, more and more researchers and scientists emphasize today.

The only question then is how and with what food?

The whole book shows you which foods will protect you from cancer or keep it at bay. In Part C, you read about how to eat healthy. This part D is like a little summary specifically related to cancer. I'm not going to add any more comments here in Part D for many foods, but just list them, because you'll find the detailed explanations in Part C.

The second prevention, but which should really be the first: Our psyche

What you should keep in mind when applying these tips is simple: listen to yourself, believe in yourself, realize that nature and the world do not mean you any harm. Your mental attitude towards cancer is the most important thing. You should never panic, because science has already made a lot of progress and you don't always and not necessarily have to die immediately because of cancer. Then, if you trust nature and use its immense treasures, you can defeat cancer, even though it may not disappear. Victory starts in the mind. If you reject that it scares and panics you, if you accept it and make contact with this foreign "body" that is now a part of you, you will undermine its threat and find the right way - because the next level of prevention when cancer has broken out is not the drugs but is your psyche.

Keep your head up if you are not sick, keep your head even higher if you are sick. Everything is in your hands. Don't give up by starting to eat healthy **now.**

D2 The sun is also "food" against cancer

The sun is not directly a food, but the sun also nourishes the body. The sun's rays stimulate the skin to produce large amounts of the cancer-inhibiting vitamin D. Vitamin D deficiency can lead to chronic diseases like cancer. Many scientific studies confirm that there is a link between vitamin D deficiency and colon, prostate or breast cancer and also one to type I diabetes, multiple sclerosis or rheumatoid arthritis. More on this in chapter D5.

It has been found that people who get little sun are more likely to develop cancer. It has been proven that artificial radiation in the tanning salon has zero healing effect and does not stimulate the body to produce vitamin D at all.

Researchers believe that solar radiation has its greatest effect on people who already have cancer.

D3 Sport can also be "food" against cancer

When I was sick as a child, my father would say to me: "Go outside for a minute and walk a little!"

I consider sports as anti-cancer "food". My father always said that a healthy mind can only live in a healthy body, and when the body is healthy, it in turn strengthens the mind. But both are nourished by diet and exercise. That is, both a healthy diet and exercise can heal. I will go further and say that exercising is also nutrition for the human being. Just like nutrition, exercise has a healing effect on cancer. Exercise or sports can prevent cancer, like a medicine. It can protect against the development of tumors and for those who are already ill, it can positively support the therapy and extend their life expectancy.

Why I consider sports as food?

This has to do with the way sport works in us, what reactions it triggers. These are almost the same reactions that some foods trigger in our body.

Sport has an effect on processes in the body that make it more difficult for cancer to develop, just like some foods. It also has a positive effect on cancer patients and supports drug therapy. There is a lot of evidence of the positive effect in relation to prostate, breast and uterine cancer. Some studies show that sport reduces the risk of cancer: for breast cancer by 20-40%, for colorectal cancer by 40-50%.

- Sport brings and generates energy
- Sport alleviates negative side effects of chemotherapy
- Sport boosts and strengthens the immune system

- Sport fights obesity and thus acts against cancer, diabetes and cardiovascular disease
- Sport can prevent relapse
- Sport lowers estrogen levels in blood and tissue, especially in women with hormone-dependent growing breast cancer. In this case, sport works even as well as drug-based, anti-hormonal therapy
- Sport has a positive effect on the psyche, which is important when you suffer from cancer
- Sport improves memory and strengthens the brain
- Sport boosts DNA repair
- Sport improves the function of the cardiovascular system
- Sport improves the fitness of the body and its resistance to diseases
- Sport accelerates detoxification
- Sport lowers the level of certain growth factors and hormones
- Sport brings tone to the cells
- Sport stimulates the metabolism
- Sport helps to lose weight and thus also lowers cholesterol levels
- Through sport, antioxidants act more effectively, respectively sport has an antioxidant effect, so free radicals are combated

It seems that the more and the more often you exercise, the more your risk of developing cancer decreases.

D3.1 Exercise and sport for breast cancer

- Avoid muscle shortening
- Improve an already existing lymphedema
- Compensate for lack of power (right-left comparison)
- Improve limited mobility (contracture prophylaxis)
- Improve overall fitness
- Combat chronic fatigue (fatigue syndrome)
- Reduce osteoporosis
- Reduce the hand-foot syndrome (polyneuropathy)
- Promotes self-esteem and thus combats the feeling of "defeminization"

(Excerpt: www.krebshilfe.de)

D3.2 Exercise and sport for prostate cancer

- Improve incontinence
- Improve the perception of the own body
- Strengthen the pelvic floor muscles
- Combat chronic fatigue (fatigue syndrome)
- Help to learn relieving postures
- Help to learn proper breathing techniques
- Improve overall fitness
- Help learn back and pelvic floor friendly everyday techniques

- Strengthen self-confidence

(Excerpt: www.krebshilfe.de)

D3.3 Exercise and sport with gastric and colorectal cancer

- Promote body awareness
- Improve mobility in the operated area
- Strengthen the trunk and back muscles
- Caution after abdominal surgery
- Stretch and strengthen the abdominal muscles (carefully)
- Improve the overall physical condition
- Builds performance for everyday life
- Improve overall fitness
- Promote self-esteem
- Strengthen self-confidence

(Excerpt: www.krebshilfe.de)

D3.4 Exercise and sport in leukemia and lymphoma diseases

- Prevent deficiency diseases (such as cardiovascular diseases) caused by too little exercise
- Combat fatigue and exhaustion
- Build muscles

- Strengthen especially the leg and back muscles
- Improve lung function
- Reduce the hand-foot syndrome (polyneuropathy)

(Excerpt: www.krebshilfe.de)

D4. The anti-cancer foods: which foods help against cancer, or prevent it?

After cardiovascular diseases, cancer is among the most common causes of death in the Western world. As with heart disease, diet plays a very important role with cancer. A first important step is to avoid milk and dairy products; you should greatly reduce your consumption of dairy products overall. Many scientific studies show that a healthy diet can prevent cancer or greatly help accompanying cancer therapy. Some of these foods are:

D4.1 Alkaline food

A balanced and even more alkaline than acidic environment is perfect for preventing cancer from developing or even suppressing it, because many alkaline foods are the source of numerous anti-cancer substances and antioxidants.

See chapter C3.9. "Alkaline food".

D4.2 Bitter foods, such as kale, broccoli and co.

In Cameroon, it is often said that good remedies taste bitter. And indeed, many natural medicines, especially in the form of drinks, are bitter. The fight against cancer often starts in our intestines. A healthy intestinal flora is important to protect against this disease and bitter foods are an excellent remedy and cleanser for the intestines.

Bitter foods stimulate digestion and it is known that poor digestion is the cause of many diseases, because it allows bacteria and viruses to emerge that also cause cancer.

Besides the already known bitter apricot kernel, other bitter foods are also good fighters against cancer. Many bitter foods contain numerous antioxidants.

See chapter C3.8. "Bitter foods".

D4.3 Anti-cancer spices and herbs

Actually, herbs should not be called food, because they are real remedies. They are the true free and healthy pharmacy of nature.

The following herbs and spices are cancer enemies:

- Ginger
- Onion
- Garlic
- Hot chili
- Parsley
- Basil
- Thyme
- Sage
- Coriander
- Rosemary
- Oregano
- Cinnamon

D4. The anti-cancer foods: which foods help against cancer, or prevent it?

- Turmeric/Curcumin
- Wormwood
- Black Seed
  "The black seeds are a cure for all diseases except death," said the Prophet Mohamed in his time.

D4.4 Anti-cancer fruit and fruits

D4.4.1 Tropical fruit

Pineapple

See chapter C3.10.6

Papaya

Papaya inhibits the growth of cancer cells and is used in Africa, green or yellow, as a powerful remedy for chronic inflammation, including cancer.

Science is slowly recognizing the benefits of this fruit in the fight against cancer. Hundreds of studies on the papaya prove its healing properties. The Australian authorities even advertise that the papaya is a cure for cancer. It is said to be effective against breast cancer as well as cervical, pancreatic and other types of cancer. This effect is explained by the numerous antioxidants found in large quantities in papaya through phenolic compounds (catéchines, beta cryptoxanthin, lycopene, papain).

Several studies have shown that increasing the consumption of foods rich in lycopene reduces the risk of prostate cancer.

ee chapter C3.10.7.

D4. The anti-cancer foods: which foods help against cancer, or prevent it?

Avocados

Avocados are said to be a miracle weapon against cancer.

Many people and naturopaths in Cameroon know that the avocado tree with its fruit is a medicinal plant that is also used to treat chronic diseases.

Now science is also recognizing the healing power of this plant and it is even said to be anticarcinogenic, according to a study from Canada. Researchers at the University of Waterloo discovered an ingredient in avocado that can fight cancer. This substance, avocatin B, is a fat that has been successful in treating acute myeloid leukemia (AML). What makes this fat special is that it fights the cancer where it originated, without attacking the healthy cells.

Although researchers say that it will be years before this fat is sold as a medicine, but the good thing is that we do not have to wait so long, because we can eat avocados at any time. Just take matters into your own hands and eat this fruit regularly from now on.

See chapter C3.10.8.

Coconut and coconut oil

Coconut oil is said to eliminate colon cancer cells, according to laboratory studies. Coconut oil contains about 50% lauric acid. This acid has destroyed up to 93% of colon cancer cells in the laboratory. You can't always transfer lab studies 1 to 1 to humans. But it is a sign for me that this food can support the body to prevent or suppress cancer and slow down its development.

See chapter C3.10.5.

Safou

This tropical fruit and its seeds contain a cytotoxic substance that is 10,000 times more effective against cancer than normal chemotherapy with the drug adriamycin, according to research published in the *Journal of Natural Products in* 1996.

See chapter C3.10.9.

Citrus fruits: grapefruit, lemons, oranges

Are among the most antioxidant fruits that eliminate free radicals.

See chapter C3.10.11.

Mango

See chapter C3.10.12.

Guava

See chapter C3.10.14

Soursop

A very effective anti-cancer agent.

See chapter C3.10.10

D4.4.2 Other fruit

Tomatoes

Tomatoes contain large amount of lycopene. It is a carotenoid which is responsible for the red color of tomatoes. Tomato is by far the best source of nutrition. Of all carotenoids, lycopene is the one with the greatest impact on cancer prevention, because it is one of the powerful antioxidants and is considered a radical scavenger. Thus, it can render reactive molecules in the human body harmless and save cells from destruction.

Several epidemiological studies have indicated that high consumption of tomatoes can protect lungs and stomach from cancer.

Pomegranate

Pomegranate juice has anti-inflammatory and antioxidant effects. Pomegranate is a fruit with many antioxidants, flavonoids, tannins and ellagic acid (40%). The activity of its antioxidants is even greater than that of green tea.

This makes the pomegranate a remedy for many chronic diseases and is also said to be effective against cancer. During various studies with pomegranate polyphenols, an inhibited growth of cancer cells in the mammary gland, lung, skin, intestine and prostate was observed, according to Wikipedia.

Berries, the darker the better

The small red fruits such as raspberries, blueberries, blackberries, etc. contain large amounts of polyphenols with the well-known anti-cancer effect.

One polyphenol that can interfere with the development of cancer is ellagic acid. It has shown a cancer-preventing effect in animal studies. Ellagic acid is reported to stop the cell division of cancer cells.

The polyphenol is present in large quantities especially in raspberries and strawberries. In raspberries, the ellagic acid is 90% in the seeds. In order that these are not excreted unchewed, because they are difficult for the organism to absorb, I would recommend to puree the whole fruit before consuming it. With strawberries it is different. The acid is found in the whole strawberry flesh.

The second type of polyphenols in berries, which are also anticarcinogenic, are anthocyanidins. They have a strong antioxidant potential. They are mostly found in blueberries and bilberries, but also in small amounts in raspberries, strawberries and cranberries.

Finally, red fruits contain proanthocyanidins, also a powerful antioxidant. In the laboratory it was found that the intake of this substance inhibits the growth of various cancer cells.

Plum

The plum contains various phenolic compounds, especially flavonoids and phenolic acids - effective antioxidants. Dried plums still contain almost the same amount of antioxidants and thus rank second among dried fruits containing antioxidants.

As prune juice, the fruit also does not lose its power as an antioxidant.

Studies in the laboratory have shown that the consumption of prunes reduced the growth of colon cancer cells.

A University of Texas study also proved the effect of plum extracts against breast cancer growth.

Peach and nectarine

Peaches and nectarines are good antioxidants because of their high content of phenolic compounds. The combination with vitamin C and carotenoids increases their antioxidant effect. These fruits reduce damage caused by oxidative stress. They have anti-inflammatory and anti-cancer effects.

Raisin (dried grape)

The raisin has one of the highest contents of antioxidants among fruits.

Apricot kernels

Apricot kernels contain vitamin B17, which has been used by some in the fight against cancer. B17 tablets with apricot kernel extract are available in Australia and the USA.

Chokeberry

A dark blue berry with scientifically proven anti-cancer effects.

D4.5 Anti-cancer vegetables

Moringa is the best vegetable not only to prevent cancer, but also to stop its spread and metastasis. With over 46 antioxidants, the moringa can fight against many types of cancer. See chapter C3.10.1.

Other vegetables are: bamboo shoots, broccoli, cabbage, chicory, cauliflower, carrots, garlic, sweet potatoes, mushrooms, beans, cassava, yam, taro leaves, bitter leaf, bean leaves, pumpkin leaves, peas, lentils, pumpkin seeds.

D4.6 Anti-cancer salads

The following salads can have a positive effect in an overall anti-cancer diet: chicory, curled lettuce, iceberg lettuce, endive, lamb's lettuce, lettuce, dandelion, lollo.

D4.7 Anti-cancer nuts

Nuts also contain important substances that can prevent cancer. Hazelnuts, Brazil nuts, walnuts, almonds, palm kernel nut, cashew nuts and small Cameroon peanuts (natural), best eaten directly from the shell when freshly harvested.

Eat nuts preferably untreated, unroasted and unsalted.

D4.8 Anti-cancer meat

Contrary to what many nutrition experts say, meat is not necessarily unhealthy. It depends. Doctors in Cameroon told me that northern Cameroonians, who eat a lot of beef, have the fewest cases of cancer. The women there have the firmest breasts, even after having several children, and breast cancer is almost unknown there.

In Cameroon, beef is very healthy. The cattle live outdoors and feed only on grass. They are almost fat-free and full of muscle. The meat tastes totally different from the meat in Europe. It's organic, totally without chemicals. It is not meat itself that is bad, but the toxins in the meat. The fact that beef is so fatty here in Europe has to do with the chemical-rich diet of cattle and the way they are fed meat meal, wheat, etc. It's not natural. Beef and venison have nutrients that are important for the body. Some studies show that controlled consumption of lean meat lowers the risk of certain cancers.

In Cameroon, offal is also considered a source of nutrients.

Instead of assessing the quality of meat, researchers condemn it completely, even though there are peoples who eat a lot of beef, but where hardly any cases of cancer are found, for example in Chad in Africa.

What if healthy beef did fight breast cancer?

D4.9 Anti-cancer fish

Marine fish inhibit cancer formation. Eating fish two to three times a week significantly reduces the risk of breast, colon and prostate cancer. Some studies even say up to almost 40%.

Suitable fish are:

Salmon, mackerel, herring and sardines.

D4.10 Anti-cancer fats

Omega fatty acids are good, but fatty acid blends (saturated and monounsaturated and polyunsaturated) are better for the healing power of an oil, especially against cancer, my teacher in Africa told me. Sometimes even, as in the case of palm oil, a higher saturated fat content can help better. More important is the overall composition of the oil.

Foods rich in omega-3 fatty acids are part of any effective anti-cancer diet. Studies have shown a link between eating fish rich in omega-3s and a lower risk of certain types of cancer such as breast, ovarian, prostate and colon cancer. But these fats are only effective against cancer when consumed through food, otherwise the effect will reverse, especially in postmenopausal women, as evidenced by a 2009 Korean study.

Omega-3 fatty acids are especially found in vegetable oils such as palm oil, olive oil, linseed oil, hemp oil, and in fish, such as salmon.

A mixture of different fatty acids makes fat an effective anticancer agent. In the Western diet, fatty acids are considered separately and in isolation. Omega-3 fatty acids are presented as the healthiest fat. But in holistic healing nutrition it does not work that way. A good composition of different fatty acids is much more important in healing diseases.

- **Palm oil**
- **Coconut oil**
- **Peanut oil**

Peanut oil is a vegetable oil made from pressed peanuts. It is a very healthy oil. Wikipedia states that the European Pharmacopoeia specifies the following fatty acid composition for the purity of refined peanut oil: 35 to 72% monounsaturated oleic acid, 13 to 43% diunsaturated linoleic acid, 7 to 16% palmitic acid, 1.3 to 6.5% stearic acid, 0.5 to 3% arachidic acid, 1 to 5% behenic acid, and 0.5 to 3% lignoceric acid. Furthermore, tocopherols (several forms of vitamin E), other antioxidants, lecithin, hydrocarbons, sterols and 13 different vitamins including A, B, C and E are found in it. A perfect blend for health. There is a difference between African peanut oil and other peanut oils. The African peanut oil is yellowish, still tastes a bit like peanut and is very healthy.

Peanut oil, because of its content of unsaturated fatty acids in the triacyl glycerides, lowers cholesterol.

This oil used to be mixed as peanut paste even in many ointments, because it has analgesic effect. It is used to relieve muscle, joint and rheumatic pains. This oil is also very helpful for skin problems and acne. The oil is also used in Africa for colds and stuffy noses and is an excellent cleanser for the intestines. It stimulates digestion, makes the intestinal flora healthy and helps the body to absorb nutrients well.

The oil is antioxidant and protects the body from free radical damage and thus from chronic diseases such as cancer. According to natural medicine experts in Cameroon, peanut oil from Africa in particular is a good preventative against cancer. Eating a tablespoon of peanut butter at least four times a week reduces the risk of cardiovascular disease and helps reduce colon cancer and Alzheimer's disease.

- **Shea butter from the tree of life**

Shea butter is a fatty oil derived from the African shea tree, also known as "The Tree of Life". Shea butter has been recognized for thousands of years for its many healing properties and uses. This is unrefined butter. Refined and highly processed butter is not as healthy and has already lost many of its nutrients.

D4. The anti-cancer foods: which foods help against cancer, or prevent it?

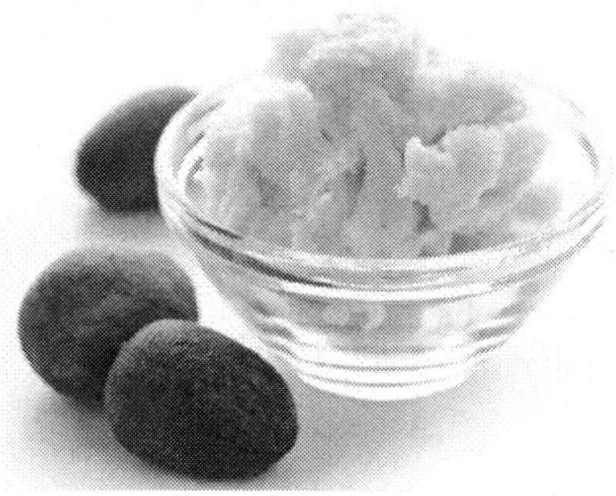

Shea butter not only helps the appearance and makes a beautiful skin, as many think, no, shea butter contains many vitamins - D, E, F - essential fatty acids and minerals. Thus, it also has an antioxidant effect and is used in Africa against chronic infections. Many natural doctors in Cameroon use shea butter to prevent or cure skin cancer.

- **Olives and olive oil**

In olive oil are antioxidants that can block the initial development of cancer. Olive oil also contains phenolic compounds. Black olives contain more than green and thus also have a greater antioxidant capacity.

Olives and olive oil have a protective effect against breast cancer, colon cancer and uterine cancer, according to studies. Cold-pressed olive oil is said to make it more difficult for metastases to form, a Canadian study said.

- **Other oils: walnut oil, linseed oil**

There is also a certain type of algae that is very rich in omega-3 fatty acids. The oil of this alga can be consumed very easily in the form of a special oil mixture together with linseed oil, evening primrose oil and other valuable ingredients.

D4.11 Anti-cancer drinks and teas

Drinks can also protect against cancer. The following teas are particularly rich in antioxidants:

- Rooibos tea
- Green tea
- Green tea with ginger
- Ginger tea (also with lemon)
- Moringa tea is great!
- Tea with cola nut powder
- Citrus juices in various compositions
- Lemon with honey, lukewarm
- Coconut milk from fresh coconut
- Coconut milk with raspberries
- Pomegranate juice
- Pomegranate juice with lemon
- Pomegranate juice with green tea
- Juice of papaya, pineapple and mango (almost like smoothies, often used by natural medicine practitioners in Cameroon against chronic infections. Sometimes the green papaya is mixed in).
- Soursop juice
- Mango juice (also with pineapple, orange and apple, etc.)
- Grape juice
- Tomato juice

D4. The anti-cancer foods: which foods help against cancer, or prevent it?

- Berry juices, such as raspberry juice
- Juice from: lemon, carrot, beet, apple. This juice is said to have a very strong anti-cancer effect. (Source for this tip: http://livefreelivenatural.com/the-miracle-drink-that-kills-cancer-cells/)
- Pineapple and ginger
- Orange and raspberry juice
- Safou juice
- Salt water with lemon and ginger: In Africa, many healers say that sea water is effective against cancer
- Garlic drinks: puree garlic and ginger, add to warm water and let rest for 48 hours. Filter and drink by the cup with lemon juice and honey. This is a super energy drink for health in general

And much more

*** Everybody says that green tea helps, but during my research I found that most women who had cancer also drank a lot of teas and green teas????

D5 The most important anti-cancer vitamins

Vitamins are good helpers against cancer. But only if they are taken in a natural way. That means through the diet. The body processes artificially produced vitamins poorly and, on the contrary, tries to defend itself against them, which further stresses the body and creates free radicals.

Artificial vitamins in tablet form as dietary supplements are dangerous for the body. They are completely overdosed, make some tumors grow properly and even make some cancer patients die earlier. The risk of cancer is even much higher if other important substances are missing at the same time. For example, taking artificial vitamin E increases prostate cancer if selenium is deficient at the same time.

That is why it is very important to absorb these vitamins from fresh foods.

- **Vitamin D, a very important hormone against cancer**

Several studies around the world have shown that vitamin D (or "calciferol") may prevent breast, prostate and colon cancer. It may also slow the development of the cancer.

Vitamin D is a fat-soluble vitamin that is produced naturally, under the influence of UV rays (sun) in the skin. Just a few hours a week in fresh air will help the body synthesize vitamin D. It is also important to go outside when the weather is bad or the sky is overcast. Because despite cloud cover, enough UV radiation still makes it to the earth's surface. Up to 90% of the required vitamin D is formed in the skin by the sun.

Vitamin D can also be absorbed to a very limited extent through food. It is mainly present in mushrooms (porcini), cod liver oil, beef liver, egg and in fish (salmon, mackerel). In the case of mushrooms, it is necessary to fry them briefly in oil, because vitamin D is fat-soluble and it is only during cooking that it develops or is better absorbed by the body.

Vitamin D is not a vitamin in the true sense, but a hormone. It was mistakenly named and assigned to the vitamins after it was found in cod liver oil and found to be able to fight rickets in children.

Vitamin D plays an important role in our health. It helps in calcium and phosphate metabolism and is thus important for bone formation. It is also involved in many metabolic processes, protects the body against infection, helps build muscle.

People who lack vitamin D have a hard time losing weight, especially in the abdominal area. A good supply of vitamin D is important if you want to lose weight. This finding is confirmed by more and more scientific studies.

Vitamin D also has an influence on the distribution of fat pads on the body: with a good vitamin D supply, belly fat is "burned" better and disappears faster. Especially for people who want to build muscles and have a six-pack, vitamin D is indispensable. Studies show that women who took in little vitamin D have a higher fat storage in the muscles.

Vitamin D deficiency can lead to chronic diseases, such as cancer. Many scientific studies confirm that there is a link between vitamin D deficiency and colon, prostate and breast cancer and also with type I diabetes, multiple sclerosis, rheumatoid arthritis.

Vitamin D deficiency can also promote osteoporosis, especially in women, but also in men (more so in the elderly); as well as rickets in children and osteomalacia in adults (bone softening).

Since vitamin D is fat soluble, it is well bound in fat and removed from the blood, so overweight people lose vitamin D (because of too much fat) and cannot store it. They end up suffering from vitamin D deficiency, which causes their parathyroid gland to stop functioning well (parathyroid overactivity). Further, they suffer from mineralization defects in the bones.

Vitamin D protects cells and protects against cancer. Weight loss, combined with vitamin D, noticeably reduces inflammation associated with cancer as well as other chronic diseases.

Vitamin D is also an excellent anti-aging agent. Perhaps it is also one of the reasons why people in Africa suffer less from cancer and have fewer wrinkles in comparison?

Attention: UV-A light from tanning salons does not lead to vitamin D formation in our body.

- **Vitamin A and provitamin A**

Thanks to its antioxidant effects, vitamin A is an anticarcinogen.

- **Vitamin C: Anti-free radicals**

Vitamin C is a powerful water-soluble antioxidant that fights free radicals very well, protecting cells and DNA from oxidative attack and destruction. It helps prevent cells from mutating. The body is protected from nasty inflammations and thus the cancer is deprived of its milieu.

- **Carotenoids**

Like vitamin C, carotenoids are very effective antioxidants and radical scavengers. They protect body substances and metabolic systems from harmful influences.

According to Wikipedia, carotenoids are an extensive class of natural pigments that cause a yellow to reddish coloration. Carotenoids belong to the terpenes. Today, 800 different carotenoids have been identified.

Carotenoids cause the red and yellow coloration in various parts of plants. But green vegetables such as spinach, peas, beans or broccoli also contain carotenoids, but they are not visible because they are hidden by the green chlorophyll of the plants. Beta-carotene represents 20 to 35% of the amount of carotenoids present in the blood.

By counteracting oxidative changes in biologically important molecules, increased carotenoid intake reduces the risk of certain types of cancer: prostate, esophageal and stomach cancer.

The carotenoids of interest are mainly beta-carotene, alpha-carotene, lycopene, lutein, zeaxanthin and cryptoxanthin.

Carotenoids are found, for example, in:

- Apricots
- Chanterelles
- Paprika
- Shrimp, lobster, salmon
- Carrots
- Kale
- Oranges
- Spinach
- Tomatoes

- **The vitamin B series: important substances against cancer.**

Vitamin B is a vitamin group with 8 vitamins (B1, B2, B3, B5, B6, B7 or vitamin H, B9 or folic acid, B12). It is found in animal foods, especially liver products and fish, and in plant foods (except vitamin B12) such as spinach, kale, broccoli, in many African foods, etc.

  - **Vitamin B9:**

A study from Sweden that lasted over 7 years and included nearly 90,000 subjects showed that vitamin B9 reduced the risk of pancreatic cancer.

Several other studies have shown that vitamin B9 could fight various types of cancer: colon cancer, breast cancer and ovarian cancer. It may also help alleviate the side effects of anti-cancer treatment.

Vitamin B9 is also believed to prevent or improve the healing of heart disease. Vitamin B9 is found in the liver of beef and poultry.

  - **Vitamin B12**

It is found especially in liver, meat, eggs, milk and algae, but hardly in plant products.

  - **Vitamin B17**

Supposed to be very effective against cancer. Many people report how they have successfully stopped cancer with vitamin B17. Many scientists doubted this theory.

I can only say that vitamin B17 has generally good properties and it can't hurt to eat healthy foods that contain it.

Vitamin B17 is found in apricot kernels.

Manioc, yam roots and leaves contain sufficient vitamin B17. Especially manioc contains a lot of this vitamin and has always been used against cancer in Cameroon. (Maybe because of this vitamin???)

Vitamin B17 can be found in:

- very small amounts in some berries: wild blackberries, elderberries, gooseberries, blueberries, strawberries, raspberries.
- the kernels of some fruits: apple, apricot, cherry, nectarine, peach, pear, plum
- some beans: mungo, fava, lentils, green peas, kidney
- nuts: macadamia, cashew, bitter almond
- leaves: eucalyptus, alfalfa, spinach
- sprouts: bamboo

I would just prefer the African version, with manioc and yam, because they contain not only vitamin B17, but also other B vitamins. They are easy to cook and taste good. I also recommend making smoothies with the fruits mentioned above.

- **Vitamin E**

Vitamin E is said to eliminate cancer stem cells and it is considered by some to be an anti-prostate cancer agent. It is strongly antioxidant and a good free radical scavenger, preventing the development of certain cancerous tumors. A 2008 study from the US highlighted the usefulness of this vitamin in preventing prostate cancer, especially in smokers.

Vitamin E can be found in vegetable oils, such as palm oil, coconut oil or olive oil and in hazelnuts, walnuts, almonds, moringa and in many African foods.

- **Vitamin K: Prevents cancer?**

A study published in the *Journal of the American Medical Association* showed that vitamin K (and specifically vitamin K2) can very successfully prevent cancer. In the study, people who showed an increased risk of liver cancer were divided into two groups. One of the groups received vitamin K2. In the end, the result was clear and very obvious: less than 10% of the subjects who received vitamin K2 later developed liver cancer. On the other hand, 47% of the control group, which did not receive vitamin K, developed liver cancer.

A German study published in 2010 in the *American Journal of Clinical Nutrition* shows a similar result. Vitamin K2 reduces the risk of cancer (prostate, lung) and prevents deaths from the cancer.

These studies are only indications, but not proof that vitamin K really prevents cancer. But since vitamins are also found in healthy foods, there is no harm in getting them in your diet.

D6 Anti-cancer minerals

- **Selenium**

According to several studies, selenium could help in the prevention of various types of cancer such as prostate, lung, bladder, and colon cancer. This trace element is one of the most powerful natural antioxidants, along with vitamins C and E and carotenoids.

It is found, for example, in cod, tuna, monkfish, herring or oysters.

- **Iron, manganese**

If one has iron and manganese in very small amounts in the body, they help eliminating free radicals that harm the body and increase the risk of cancer. In addition, manganese also promotes the production of vitamin E, a powerful antioxidant.

D7 Essential fatty acids and oils against breast cancer?

Our body cannot produce essential fatty acids itself, which is why they have to be taken in through food. Serious malnutrition can occur if the body is not supplied with sufficient essential fatty acids. These long-chain, polyunsaturated fatty acids are vital for our body.

Deficiency of essential fatty acids can harm the body and cause many diseases. The deficiency can also lead to chronic diseases and infections, migraine and depression, hormonal imbalances, skin changes and hair loss.

Essential fatty acids ensure that transport processes, such as that of oxygen, and other functions can be carried out in the cell membranes. They thus contribute to the construction and maintenance of cell walls.

Naturopaths in Cameroon recommend these fatty acids to prevent chronic diseases, especially breast, colon and prostate cancer. The oil is mixed with some other substances (including ginger) and women are supposed to massage their breasts with it or/and drink a spoonful of it every morning and evening. This is even said to suppress cancer that has already developed. Also, many scientific studies suggest that there may be a connection between certain types of cancer and deficient vegetable oils. These oils supply the breast with important nutrients and enough oxygen and catch free radicals. This way, they help to prevent cell damage from occurring in the first place, and if it does, to repair it quickly or reactivate the cell.

Either way, even without 100% scientific proof, there's no harm in consuming a little good oil in your diet. It can only help.

Essential fatty acids consist exclusively of the doubly unsaturated linoleic acid and the triply unsaturated alpha-linolenic acid. These are found almost exclusively in plant foods and vegetable oils (linseed oil, coconut oil, peanut oil, palm oil, safflower oil, soybean oil, sunflower oil, walnut oil, wheat germ oil).

The use of oils as a healing agent has been practiced in Africa for thousands of years.

D8 Which foods against which type of cancer?

Depending on the type of cancer, is there a very special way to eat? Certain foods that only fight certain types of cancer?

Reading through the literature, studying scientific studies and natural teachings, I find that from a nutritional perspective, it doesn't make much difference which type of cancer is present. True, some types of cancer emphasize this or that more than others, but in the end, for the purposes of this book, you should look at everything holistically. I wouldn't particularly separate from a holistic perspective. It may be that it is different for medicines and medicinal plants, but the basis of healing through nutrition is the same for all cancer types. Sure, breast cancer requires more essential fatty acids than other types of cancer. But these fatty acids always help and never harm, even if you do not suffer from breast cancer. Those who eat a generally healthy diet, eat good and, above all, suitable foods and engage in sporting activities, reduce the risk of developing cancer - of any kind. Those who already suffer from the disease will help themselves in general if they fundamentally change their diet with the tips contained in this book to slow the spread of cancer or perhaps even suppress the cancer.

D9 African-inspired cooking recipes for a week: food that heals

The following African-inspired cooking recipes are specifically Cameroonian recipes that I personally know and cook often.

Basically, Cameroonian cuisine includes many herbs and spices: Ginger, garlic, onion, chili peppers should not be missing. In addition, depending on the sauce, basil, parsley, leek and more. As you will see in a moment, the Cameroonian cuisine contains over 90% only healthy foods, which are also known for their healing properties.

Having a varied and balanced diet is important. My cooking recipes, with their combination of different foods that have an anticarcinogenic effect, target different processes associated with tumor control, thus increasing their effectiveness against cancer. The joint action is always stronger than an isolated action.

In this entire nutritional concept, exceptions with "not that healthy foods" are also allowed, because they no longer take on any significance. This way, you are also allowed to "sin" in a healthy way without harming yourself. Very strict and hard dietary changes can also harm you, especially mentally, which in turn has an impact on your health. Knowing that the psyche also plays a big role in cancer, you can understand why you should eat healthy, but also enjoy the food.

All the following dishes, from Monday to Sunday, can also be prepared without meat and fish. In my detailed manual about cancer and its fight you will find an extra chapter with some Cameroonian meals that are purely vegetarian and vegan, because the normal Cameroonian eats everything: he is a meat eater, vegetarian and vegan at the same time. According to the motto: Man is one, man is holistic.

As you will see, the daily diet of the average Cameroonian is full of strength and energy, contrary to the Western assumption of how one should eat, and Cameroonians are more muscular, stronger and fat free. People in Cameroon eat hot meals twice a day on average and in the evening, the family comes together to eat.

My African recipes are African. In Cameroon, I have never seen anyone cook like in a Western cookbook, with exact quantities. That's the best way, I think, because cooking is like art. You do it by instinct. That means you're in it yourself, you're in the center of it, so you can mix your ideas into it. How much salt do you use, how spicy should your food be? How much oil do you need? You decide that yourself. Here I give you only a framework and the rest you do yourself. Always use large quantities of onion, ginger, garlic and other herbs. They are, as I said, excellent remedies. For your healing dishes you should use at least 150g of onion, 100g of ginger and 5 big cloves of garlic.

All African meals can also be cooked vegetarian or vegan. For this, simply leave fish or meat aside. All other ingredients are fully vegetarian and vegan.

Monday:

Spinach, fried with salmon and noodles (or fried plantain)

Ingredients:

- Fresh or frozen spinach leaves or young spinach, chopped. Attention: no seasoned spinach or spinach with cream.
- Ginger, onion, garlic, chili peppers (habaneros), spring onion, leek, parsley, basil, 1 tomato
- Salmon fillet with skin
- Ripe, sweet plantain or noodles
- Oil, salt, organic vegetable broth

Preparation:

1. Wash and drain spinach (feel free to chop). You can use frozen spinach directly or let it defrost
2. Season salmon with a little salt and pepper
3. Put oil in a pan and heat. The heat does not need to be strong, less than medium. Then put in the salmon, sear both sides briefly, turn off the heat and leave in the oil for a few minutes, then remove.
4. Cut onions and add to the preheated pan with the oil of the fried salmon, along with ginger and the vegetable broth powder.

5. When the onions have browned a bit, add the spinach, stirring constantly. Now simmer for a few minutes without adding water.
6. Add the fresh tomato, chili pepper, spring onions, parsley and garlic, fry some more and add a little salt.
7. Then chop the basil and put it in, immediately turn off the heat, put the salmon in the pan, and leave it on the stove plate with the lid on.
8. Cook the pasta and eat it with the delicious vegetable salmon.

   If you want the meal to be even healthier without wheat, then instead of noodles, fry plantain or boil in water like potatoes.

Fry plantain

Suitable plantains are those that have already turned yellow. They are then sweet and, if they are very yellow, can even be eaten like normal banana. But they taste totally different from banana, even if they look similar.

Peel the sweet yellow plantain with a knife. Then cut the fruit into slices of about 0.5 cm or cut the fruit in half lengthwise and then cut into pieces of about 5 cm, lightly salt if you want.

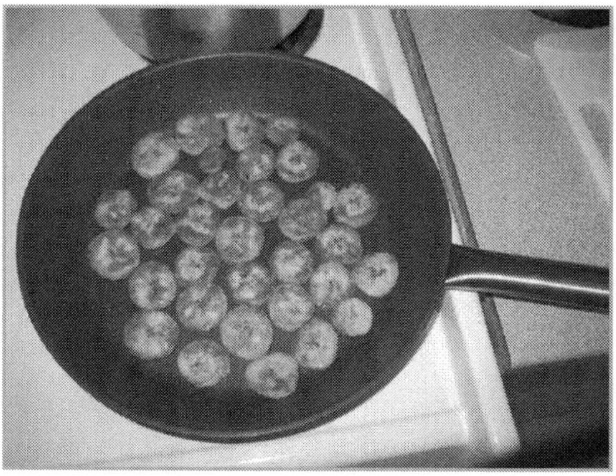

Put enough oil in the pan and when it is hot (medium, it doesn't have to be very hot), throw in the plantains and keep switching sides until they are brown, then they are done. Take them out and eat them like that or with the vegetables or with avocados or other sauces.

You can also use unsweetened plantains, the green ones, if you want.

Cooking plantain

Green plantains taste like potatoes afterwards. Yellow plantains taste sweet.

Simply peel the plantains, cut them into two or three pieces or take the whole banana, put it in a pot of salted water and cook for about 25 minutes.

Two plantains are enough for one person.

Tuesday:

Pumpkin seed sauce with fish/beef and yam

Ingredients:

- Dry pumpkin seeds from Africa: they are white (not the dark variety that you find in supermarkets. In Afro shops you can get these special, nutrient-rich, seeds, also in ground form).
- Ginger, onion, garlic, chili peppers (habaneros), 2 fresh tomatoes
- A fish of your choice or even beef
- Yam, about 350g for one person
- Oil, salt, organic vegetable broth

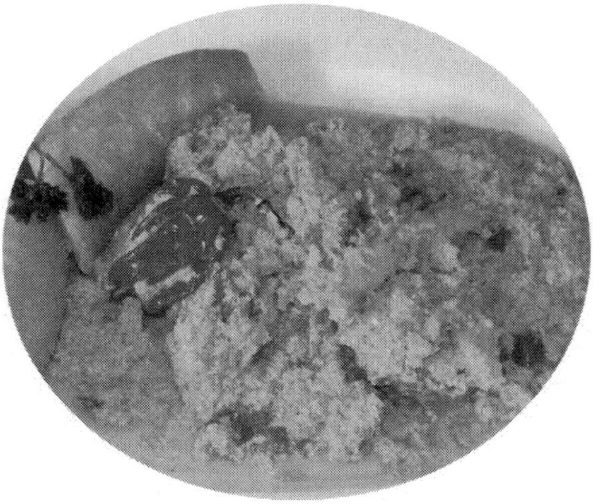

Pumpkin seed sauce with plantain

Preparation:

1. Grind pumpkin seeds in a food processor until they become a paste. You can also buy the finished paste in Afro shops
2. Season fish with a little salt and pepper or cut the meat into smaller pieces, as big as you like
3. Pour oil into a pot and heat. The heat does not have to be strong, less than medium. Then fry the fish in it and take it out again. But you do not have to fry the fish, you can just put it in the finished sauce towards the end and cook it for about 5-10 minutes at low temperature.

   If you prefer to use meat, point 3 is no longer applicable. You go directly to point 4.
4. Chop onions and toss them with ginger and garlic in the preheated pan with the oil from the fried fish.

   If you want to cook with beef, first gently roast the beef in oil briefly, then add onions, garlic, ginger and salt
5. When the onions have browned a bit, add pureed tomatoes with fresh chili and stir constantly, then pour water, close the pot and cook for about 20 minutes.
6. Then add the finely ground pumpkin seeds, reduce the heat and cook for another 25 minutes until the water has evaporated a bit and the meat is tender. You can also add water again and cook some more if the meat needs more time. If you want, add broth.
7. If the meat is okay for you, wait a little longer until the water evaporates and you start to see oil. The sauce will be

completely white. The water above the white paste should not be higher than 2 cm. Your sauce is ready.

8. Before, after or while the sauce is cooking, cook yam. Peel yam like potatoes. Cut into about 3-4 pieces and just boil like potato in salted water for about 15-20 minutes. Drain water and that's it. Add sauce and enjoy.

Wednesday:

Kale with unroasted almonds (peanuts) and plantains. National dish in Cameroon

Ingredients:

- Almonds or fresh, dried, unroasted peanuts from Afro shops. You can also use the finely ground almonds directly
- Frozen kale, defrosted
- Ginger, onions, garlic, chili peppers (habaneros), 3 fresh tomatoes, leek, spring onions, parsley
- A fish of your choice or even beef (feel free to use pork today).
- Yellow plantains: 2 per person
- Oil, salt, organic vegetable broth

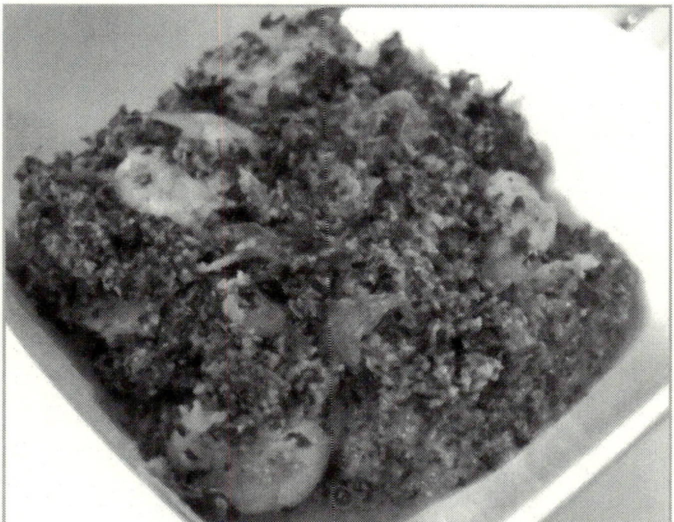

Preparation:

1. Boil almonds or peanuts in water, about 30 minutes. Remove the brown skin and then finely puree the white kernels (or directly the pre-ground almonds) with water in a food processor to a paste.
2. Boil kale briefly and squeeze out water.
3. Season fish with a little salt and pepper or cut the meat into smaller pieces, as big as you like.
4. Pour oil into a pot and heat. The heat does not have to be strong, less than medium. Then fry the fish in it and take it out again. But you do not have to fry the fish, you can just put it in the finished sauce towards the end and cook it for about 5-10 minutes at low temperature.

   If you prefer to cook with meat, then point 4 is obsolete. You go directly to point 5.
5. Cut onions and add them to the preheated pan with the oil of the fried fish, along with ginger and garlic.

   If you wanted to cook with beef, first gently roast the beef in oil briefly, then add onions, garlic, ginger and salt

   Here, many Cameroonians also do it differently. They puree all the ingredients - onions, chili, spices, herbs and fresh tomatoes - together, except for parsley, leek and spring onion. This is healthier and the nutrients are well absorbed by the body.
6. When the onions have browned slightly, add the pureed mixture (or all the chopped herbs and spices including fresh

chili), stir constantly for a few minutes, then add water, close the pot and cook for about 30 minutes.

7. Then add the fine ground paste, spring onions, leek and parsley, a little water, reduce heat and cook for another 25 minutes until the water has evaporated a little and the meat is tender. You can also add water again and cook some more if the meat needs more time. If you want, add broth.
8. When the meat is okay for you, add the kale to the white mixture in the pot, stirring constantly. Wait a bit more until the water has evaporated and you start to see oil. The delicious kale sauce is white and green. Your sauce is ready.

   Before, after or while the sauce is cooking, cook plantain.

   Green plantains taste like potatoes afterwards. Yellow plantains taste sweet.

   Simply peel the plantains, cut them into two or three pieces or take the whole plantain, put it in a pot of salted water and cook for about 25 minutes.

   Two plantains are enough for one person.

   Fried plantains also go very well with it, you are welcome to add potatoes, rice, etc. - as you like.

Thursday:

Djansang in tomato, chicken and manioc

Ingredients:

- Djansang seeds are available in Afro shops
- Ginger, onions, garlic, chili peppers (habaneros), 4 fresh tomatoes, leek, spring onions, parsley
- Chicken meat (whether leg, fillet, wings, etc., you decide)
- Manioc, about 400 g per person
- Oil, salt, organic vegetable broth

Preparation:

1. Grind djansang seeds. Per person about 10-20 pieces.
2. Season chicken to your liking
3. Pour oil into a pot and heat. Then fry chicken briefly - about 10 minutes. (But you don't have to fry the chicken, you can just add it to the sauce later and cook it).
4. Cut onions and add to the pot where the chicken is roasted.
5. When the onions are slightly brown, add all the finely chopped herbs and spices including fresh chili, stir constantly for a few minutes and then add the finely chopped tomatoes. Close the pot and cook for a few minutes.
6. Then add the finely ground djansang seeds and simmer for about 5 minutes. Refine with broth. The delicious, simple and healthy sauce is ready.

7. Before, after or while the sauce is cooking, boil manioc.

   Simply peel the manioc like potatoes, cut into two or three pieces, boil in a pot of salted water until white, about 20-30 minutes.

   Rice, noodles, potatoes, plantains and much more also go well with it.

Friday:

Macabo stew with palm oil and dried fish

Ingredients:

- Macabo root, available in Afro shops (or yam or plantain (green) as a substitute).
- Ginger, onions, garlic, chili peppers (habaneros)
- Dried and smoked fish such as mackerel, trout, salmon
- Palm oil, salt

Preparation:

1. Peel the macabo, about 400 g per person, cut into large pieces, the size of an average potato.
2. Put the pieces in a pot. Add all the pureed ingredients (or add the chopped ingredients), enough oil and water, salt and cook everything together. Always add water if necessary, until the macabo is done like a potato (about 30-45 minutes).

   Just before the end, add the smoked fish and turn off the fire. Keep the pot closed for another 15 minutes. Let water evaporate. Some like to have a lot of liquid in it, others let the water evaporate until all you see is oil, with a little water. As one likes.

   *** Cook smoked fish from Africa from the beginning. Because in this method the fish are smoked very dry.

Saturday:
Plantain porridge with kidney beans and palm oil

Ingredients:

- Fresh yellow sweet plantains, 2-3 pieces per person.
- Canned kidney beans (dry red beans, soaked in water beforehand and then cooked, would be better. This is healthier)
- Chili
- Oil, salt

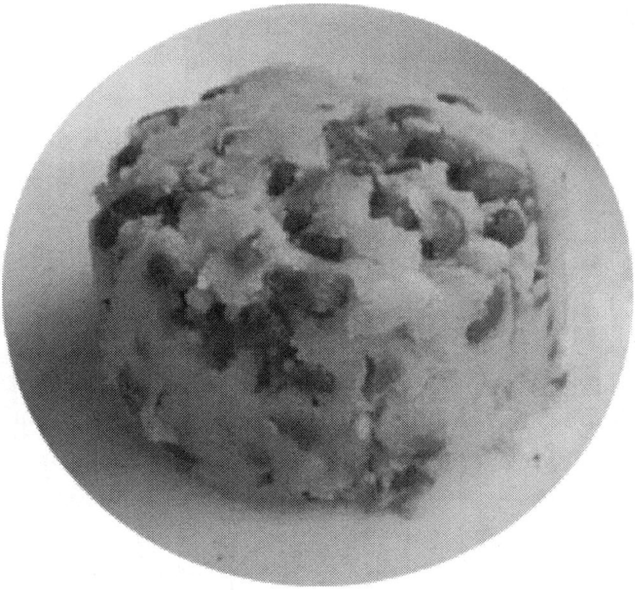

Preparation:

1. Wash the plantains well, cut them in half crosswise and boil them, including the peel, in a pot of water. If the pot is large enough, leave the plantains whole and cook them that way.
2. After about 25-30 minutes, add the kidney beans and shortly after turn off the heat.
3. Drain the water and separate the plantains from the beans.
4. Remove the skin from the plantains and mash them while still warm in a mortar, if you have one, otherwise it works in a normal pot. You can also puree everything in a blender.

   Add palm oil and chopped chili peppers and continue mashing. Then add the beans. Stir with a wooden spoon until everything is mixed. Salt. The very tasty and healthy meal without any animal additives is ready.

   Warning: it's so delicious you don't want to stop.

Sunday:

Okra sauce with fufu from manioc or dumplings

Ingredients:

- Fresh green okra from Afro or Asian shops. 250g per person
- Ginger, onions, garlic, chili peppers (habaneros), spring onions, leek
- Salmon or meat
- Manioc (fresh), or manioc flour
- Oil, salt, organic vegetable broth

Preparation:

1. Fresh okra is cut into small pieces and lightly pureed with a blender. This is how they taste best to me. I puree only briefly so they look like very heavily chopped okra. Some, however, puree them until they become slimy. Everyone, as they like.
2. Season fish with a little salt and pepper or cut the meat or even chicken into smaller pieces, as big as you like.
3. Pour oil into a pot and heat. The heat does not have to be strong, less than medium. Then put the fish in, fry it and take it out again. But you do not have to fry the fish, you can just put it in the finished sauce towards the end and cook it for about 5-10 minutes at low temperature.

   If you prefer to use meat, point 3 is no longer applicable. You go directly to point 4.

4. Cut onions and add them to the preheated pot with the oil of fried fish, along with ginger, garlic and the other ingredients and vegetable broth powder.

   If you want to cook with beef, first fry beef in oil briefly, then add onions, garlic, ginger and salt.

5. When the onions have browned slightly, add pureed tomatoes (I like to use chopped tomatoes) with fresh chili, stir constantly and then cook with a little water for about 20 minutes. (If using beef, possibly use more water and cook longer or cook the meat separately beforehand. Then it goes faster). Before adding the okra, there should not be much water.

6. After 20 minutes, add the chopped okra and keep the pot covered. After about 5 minutes, remove the lid and cook the sauce for about 15 more minutes at a mild temperature, stirring constantly, until the water is just slightly visible above the okra. Season to taste with salt and turn off the heat.

7. Fufu

   From fresh manioc: Cut into pieces, boil for about 20 minutes and pound in a mortar or puree with a blender until a viscous mass is formed. Then, using your hand, shape the mass into small portions, like a tennis ball. They will look like thicker dumplings. They are ready. Eat with the sauce.

   From manioc flour: manioc flour looks like potato flour and is prepared a bit like semolina porridge or rice pudding. Boil water in a pot. Divide the boiled water. Put one part in another container. Slowly add the flour to the water in the pot in a 2:1 ratio (two cups of water and one cup of manioc flour), stirring constantly with a wooden cooking spoon. The heat, after the water had boiled, must be quite mild so that it does not burn. Add a little water at a time and keep stirring until you have a firm, viscous mass that no longer smells of flour. Then form small dumplings and it's ready. Eat with the sauce.

You can also eat normal German dumplings with the sauce. It tastes very delicious.

You can also experiment further with potatoes.

Fried kale

You can roast kale the same way you roast spinach from Monday's recipe. It tastes very good with everything.

Boil and drain (squeeze) kale beforehand.

Soups

- Pumpkin soup with sweet potatoes and carrots, turmeric (pure), pepper, oil, ginger, salt, green tea, chili (habaneros).

  The typical anti-cancer dose of turmeric is about 3 grams of a good turmeric extract consumed three to four times a day. The problem is that turmeric is not that easily and well absorbed by the body. To avoid this problem, you should mix and blend turmeric powder and add pepper.

- Mango soup with sweet potatoes, ginger, garlic, onions, salt, chili (habaneros), oil.
- Okra, yam, lots of ginger, turmeric, lots of garlic, lots of onions, coconut oil, pepper, salt, chili (habaneros), salmon if you like.
- Peanut soup: olive oil, chili (habaneros), peanut butter with small chunks, vegetable broth, large onions, chopped garlic cloves, black pepper.
- From Dr Béliveau: garlic, Brussels sprouts, beet, cranberries, green onion, broccoli, spinach, green beans, grapefruit (100 g), turmeric in linseed oil (2 tsp turmeric mixed with 10 ml linseed oil), 6 cups green tea (2g green tea leaves to 6 cups water), black pepper (2 tsp).

Makossa hot rotic, the magic hot sauce with ginger, garlic, onion and more

No sauce has ever tasted so delicious. Eat it once and get addicted. Strengthens the body against many ailments and helps losing weight.

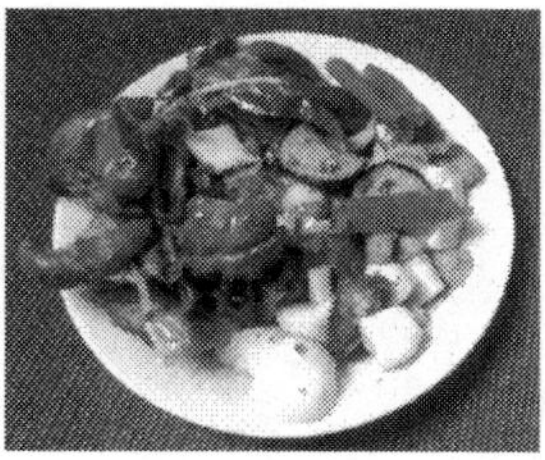
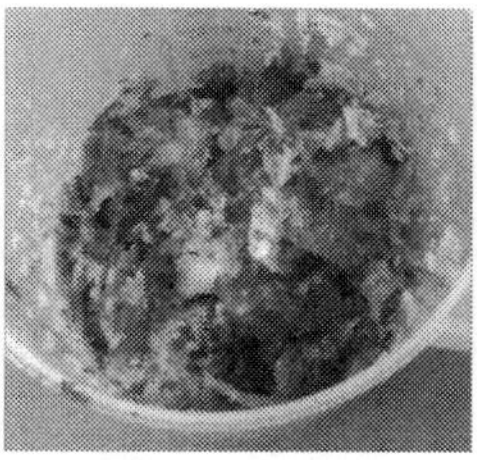
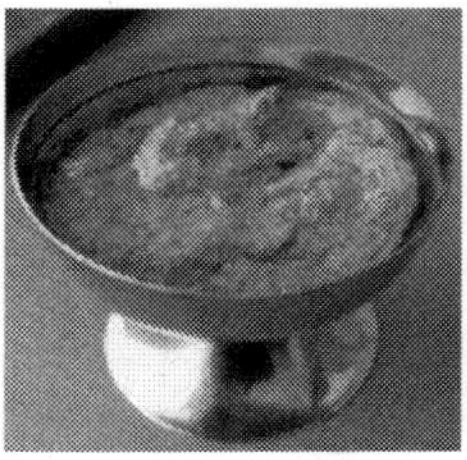

This is a wonderful sauce that was originally intended as a potency enhancing sauce but it is also very good for weight loss. The sauce is a mixture of selected potency enhancing herbs. Natural, without chemicals, preservatives and flavor enhancers! Stimulates, makes you want to have sex, promotes blood circulation, the body becomes warmer and more excited. Not only helpful for potency disorders, the sauce has an antibiotic effect and very good for fighting or preventing cancer, but also a real delicacy with meat, fish, cheese, white bread, rice, pasta, etc. Eaten regularly you will feel a lasting result and a general well-being. This sauce should no longer be missing from your menu! Effective for both men and women!

Ingredients: about 30% fresh ginger (preferably organic quality and as fresh and juicy as possible, not fibrous), about 25% onions, garlic, fresh yellow, red or green habanero chilies (very, very hot, so be careful when preparing! You can find them in Asia or Afro shops, sometimes also in well-stocked supermarkets with deli department), spring onions, lots of fresh basil, hot chili powder, fresh ramson (if available), fresh parsley, dried lovage (available in spice stores, sometimes also in tea stores), salt, organic stock powder, oil (I use normal vegetable oil, you can also use olive oil if you like it).

Preparation:

Boil lovage briefly in water and let stand for about 1-2 hours. Chop herbs and spices (important: do not peel ginger!) and puree together with the drained lovage to a paste. Mix thoroughly in a screw-top jar with plenty of oil; finally, add enough oil so that the paste is completely covered by a 1-2cm layer of oil (important for shelf life). Can be stored in the refrigerator for several weeks.

Caution: Your body will probably have to get used to the spiciness, so either increase the spiciness level slowly or consume only small amounts of the sauce at a time - otherwise you may experience gastrointestinal problems.

Tip: This sauce is also suitable as a dip for everything and can be eaten with bread, meat, cheese and so on.

With such natural remedies, no generally applicable dosage recommendation can be given, everyone must find their individual dosage. Basically, the effect is of course always related to the amount taken, i.e., a lot helps a lot (but as said: increase the degree of spiciness slowly!).

Do you have questions about the preparation? Then just message me and I'll help you with great tips.

About the author

Be different, see different, act different, so that something refreshing comes in.

My name is Dantse Dantse, I am a native of Cameroon and father of five children, some of whom are already studying. My hobbies are writing, jogging, dreaming and admiring and loving God and everything he has done.

As the oldest son of an African "troop" of 8 children of my mother and the third oldest son and seventh of all children of my late father, who had a total of 25 children with three officially married wives, my life has always been an exciting movie since I was a child. All the children and all the wives lived together in one compound, the children in one house and the father and his wives in a separate house. We all ate together, played together. One woman cooked for all the children. We children always had a contact person, because every single woman was our mother. If your own mother was away, the other mother took care of you. One has to have that experience. It's special, you learn to share, to love, with 24 equal others. Automatically, the definition of important values, such as giving, sharing, feelings, love, jealousy, patience, showing understanding, etc. is different from children of a so-called "normal" family. When you come from such a family as I did, you learn so many things that will help you in life. You learn a lot because you have to learn fast in order not to fall down.

My life continued excitingly into adulthood, not only because I am the father of five children by different, beautiful women from different cultures, but also because I have had borderline experiences, good or bad, that have shaped me. I have lost many people and gained many. I have experienced so many beautiful things, but also very painful experiences. I have tried almost everything in my life, because I am a person who is constantly looking for the new and is not afraid of risks, who is ready to go to the end to know what will become of something.

Women have always been my passion, even today, although no longer in these quantities. I had always been a little star, my star. I didn't need the success of Robbie Williams to catch on with women. Women have thus shaped my life a lot. The important thing is that I have not lost myself, but on the contrary, I have constantly evolved. Many know me as someone who thinks and lives unconventionally, who is very positive, who is a good father, for whom freedom (inner and outer) is fundamentally important, who believes in the good in people, despite some unpleasant incidents, who is helpful and likes to forgive, in short, as a person who is happy as it is, but still goes on.

A lot happened professionally, from my studies until today. I've done different things and I haven't always paid attention to the general conditions, because they usually put the brakes on. I have been living and working in Germany for over 25 years and today I work as a success coach and marketing consultant. I advise people and companies when they don't know how to go on! Before coaching, there were, as I said, many other things: studies, managing director, foreign trade, company founder, Internet, PR, and many more...

I had the idea to write when I was a child, but it was the experience I gained from my work as a consultant and coach that led me to put my hobby into practice. Since my African-inspired coaching is appealing to and helping more and more Germans, I decided, on the advice of a client, to pass on my experiences and advice in books.

My enthusiasm for everything that has to do with people is almost self-evident:

1. For 23 years I have been a father and educator of several children from different cultural backgrounds, African and European. This makes raising each child different and exciting for me as a father, but also challenging. Through these children I have also met many other children and parents.
2. Through my upbringing I learned that values and personality are very important. My father, who was very active professionally as a politician and high official of the country, always found time on weekends to tell us stories and teach us songs. We would sit for hours in the dark on the lawn in front of our houses (the parents' house and the children's house) and listen to him, his story always had to do with something that concerned us or that would strengthen us as individuals. He could tell a heartfelt story from a quote from the Bible. Those stories are still in my head decades later. In Africa, they say only a strong person as an individual makes a strong society. The other way around is unhealthy. The society would be strong, but the people in it would be broken and sick. That is why every child should seek and find his or her own way and not always bow to the dictates of the general public. Standing alone does not mean that the others are right and on the side of truth just because they are many. You can be right and

they all are not. You should not be afraid to take the path that no one else takes. You can call it a special way. But your way is the right way for you.

Children, my father said, must be brought up with values and love for self-reliance and independence. Children must be educated so that they can separate the good from the bad on their own, can recognize what is good for them, so that they can also do good for society. Children must be brought up to be happy and have the confidence that even after difficult times, which always come in a person's life, they will still continue to be happy.

Such teaching accompanied me and with time I also became more and more convinced that this is important. We see in Western countries how society is strong, but many people are weak and sick.

In such an extended family, you have to develop certain qualities and strategies to draw attention to yourself without harming the others. Many things that occupy you a lot happen at a very early age, among which the struggle for justice and equality between all the siblings towards the parents is very important. Since your parents don't have as much time for you as in a family with only two children, you have to be very attentive and solve some of your problems on your own. This means that even as a child you are a philosopher, psychologist and therapist.

As the eldest son, according to the African culture, I had to practically take over the function of an educator (here father and mother) very early. I was also specially trained for this. The best thing about this was that the oldest children were trained to be gender-neutral, so that they could take on the function of daddy and mommy at the same time. That means I've been dad and mom since I was 10. And today I'm very happy to have had those experiences and that I had the chance to co-parent my younger siblings and learn a lot from them for myself. All of this has helped me a lot in raising my own children. I learned a lot from these experiences and gained a lot of knowledge that you can hardly learn from books.

3. As a coach and consultant, I have coached many people, women, men, couples, children from different continents, cultures, social and professional circles.

   I write as I am. I write versatile, because my life is also versatile and has not taken a "normal and usual and scheduled" way, as people are used to it. I never wanted it to be that way either. I was and am the kind of person usually called a connoisseur of the art of living. Unconventional, free in my person and in my way of thinking, independent of the established, but which I fully respect. My values are love, justice, forgiveness, goodwill, optimism, generosity, responsibility, freedom with myself and with others, and being a good father.

Almost all my books are based on true events. I write books about modern issues that move people and society, books about heavy fates, taboo subjects, ethics and morals, about education, about happiness. I also write advice books and children's books with intercultural background, because my children live in intercultural circumstances. I bring experiences from two different cultures, which I had to unite in order to give my children the best possible.

This knowledge and experience has always been a great asset to people who have sought my advice.

My African-inspired tips and tricks help in all areas of life from raising children to partnership, sexuality, health, nutrition and happiness. Even the hardest nuts can be softened, with love, patience, consistency and justice. For this it is very important to know yourself, to love and to educate yourself to be happy.

My writing style is authentic and pleasant to read. The choice of words is simple, uncomplicated, understandable as well as clear. My books should make curious and thoughtful and awaken fun and desire to read. I definitely want to keep my style so that readers know me this way, accept me this way, and also recognize through it that I am not a native German. That is my incentive to write in German.

Read my books and you will understand what I have written about myself. We can continue to argue, discuss, debate and make peace. I also like to read your praise.

My author page is: www.dantse-dantse.com,

Email: Leser@dantse-dantse.com

My coaching site is: www.mycoacher.jimdo.com,

E-mail: mycoacher@yahoo.de

About indayi edition

A dream turned into an idea and the idea turned into a publishing house: indayi edition, the first FAIR publishing house!

Fair to the authors
fair literature
for a fair world

indayi edition was founded by Dantse Dantse in Darmstadt, Germany, in 2015 and is thus the first publishing house of a migrant from Africa in Germany. Dantse is originally from Cameroon and has lived in Germany for over 25 years, where he also studied. Writing books has long been his passion, and with the number of books he has published, the desire to have his own publishing house grew, so that he could remain true to his style and unconventional manner and write and publish independently of publishing guidelines and rules.

We would like to promote unconventional literature. Everything that can help people is published by us, even if it is not a trendy topic at the moment or is even taboo. In addition, literature by people with a migration background is close to our hearts - their reports on their experiences, novels, stories, recipes, their view of society, of current issues, of "the Germans", their humor and their culture. Our goal is to publish books that serve to promote understanding between cultures and that help people to better understand the world and themselves. Good, unconventional books that do not conform to the mainstream, but have topics that help society.

The books from indayi are different

...because we do not treat topics superficially, but get to the bottom of things

...because our authors write in an authentic, simple and readable way and do not use technical jargon

...because we are interested in the foreign and try to present it as it really is - unadorned and without prejudice, so that the reader feels as if he/she is there with us

...because our books solve problems and give people support, hope and motivation and also give them a smile

...because we give people with a migration background a voice

...because we use the German language for integration and peace between cultures

...because all our children's books are illustrated by children and not by professionals – this way, we show how children see the world and the stories

We want to give a voice to those who otherwise have none. The experiences, dreams, ideas, fantasies, wisdom of people with a migration background, their insights into their world open up new, unusual perspectives for us and enrich us, just like the texts of other, unconventional, lateral-thinking authors.

indayi wants to publish funny, thoughtful, philosophical, erotic, helpful, moving, touching, interesting, exciting, entertaining, controversial, insightful, amusing, amazing literature.

Visit our website: indayi.de

Subscribe to our newsletter to stay up to date:
https://indayi.de/newsletter/

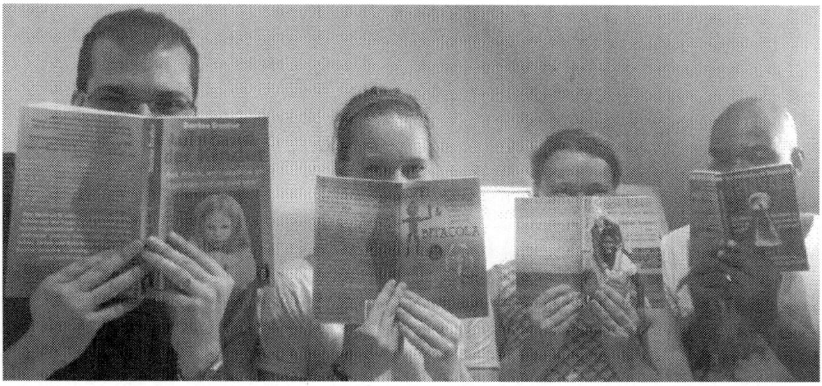

The team of indayi edition!

DIFO - DANTSE IMMUN FORTE
Life & health protect energy sauce

The therapeutic magical health sauce made from ginger, garlic, onion, chili and much more. A sauce that heals physical and mental illnesses and tastes magical. The wonderful hot sauce fights diseases very effectively and also helps losing weight.

A real delicacy with meat, fish, cheese, white bread, rice, pasta, etc. Eaten regularly, you will feel a lasting result and general well-being. This sauce should never be missing from your menu! It will never be missing once you try it for the first time!

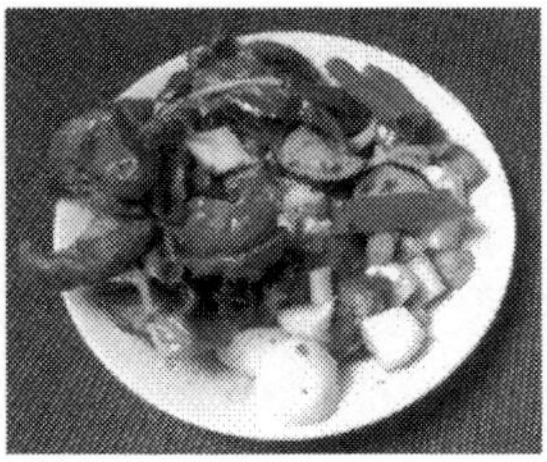

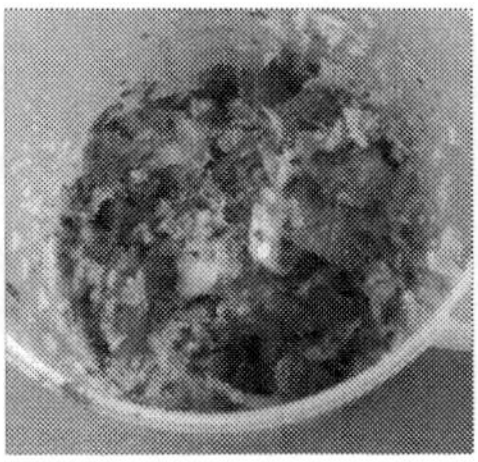

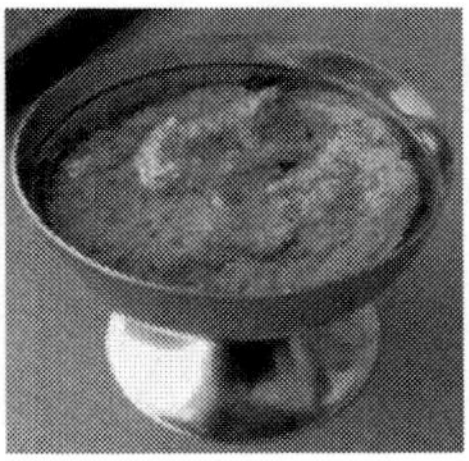

Would you like to order this sauce? Then visit www.mycoacher.jimdo.com!

DIFO Immune Formula,

contributes to the normal functioning of the immune system.

(contains vitamins A, B and C, sodium, calcium, potassium, magnesium, silicon, sulfur, phosphorus, iodine, iron, zinc)

DIFO protects your body from pathogens and helps you to **recover faster** from all diseases.
To keep your immune system strong, I recommend DIFO®:

- With the unique "Vital Formula" made from proven plants
- With the power of nature
- Contains important minerals that protect cells from oxidative stress
- Already contains the daily dose of vitamin C, A and more
- Contains important amino acids

DIFO, the delicious therapeutic sauce for optimal metabolism harmonization.

Further books by the author at indayi edition (excerpt)

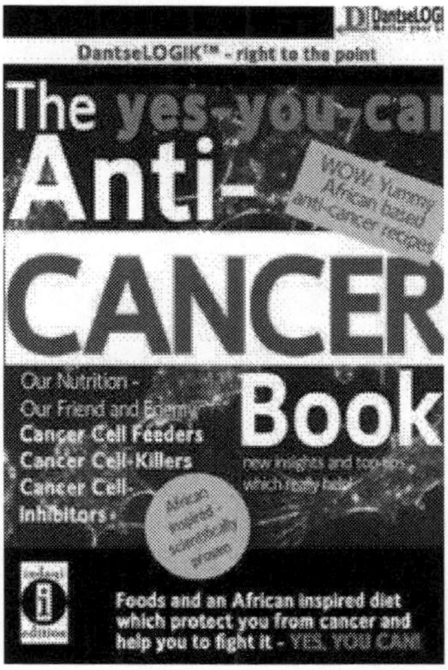

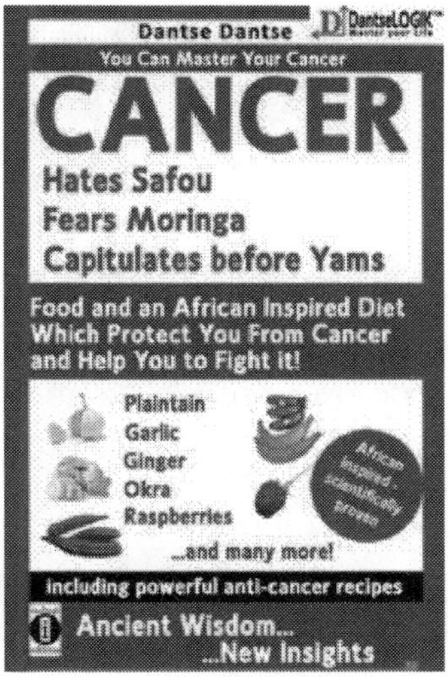

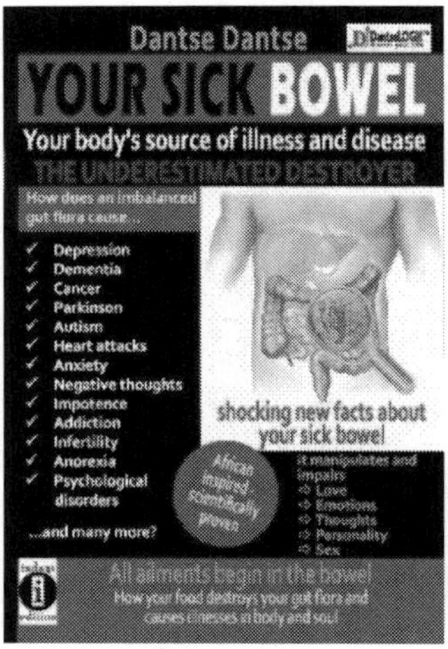
Dantse Dantse
YOUR SICK BOWEL
Your body's source of illness and disease
THE UNDERESTIMATED DESTROYER
How does an imbalanced gut flora cause...
Depression
Dementia
Cancer
Parkinson
Autism
Heart attacks
Anxiety
Negative thoughts
Impotence
Addiction
Infertility
Anorexia
Psychological disorders
...and many more?
shocking new facts about your sick bowel
African inspired scientifically proven
it manipulates and impairs
Love
Emotions
Thoughts
Personality
Sex
All ailments begin in the bowel
How your food destroys your gut flora and causes illnesses in body and soul
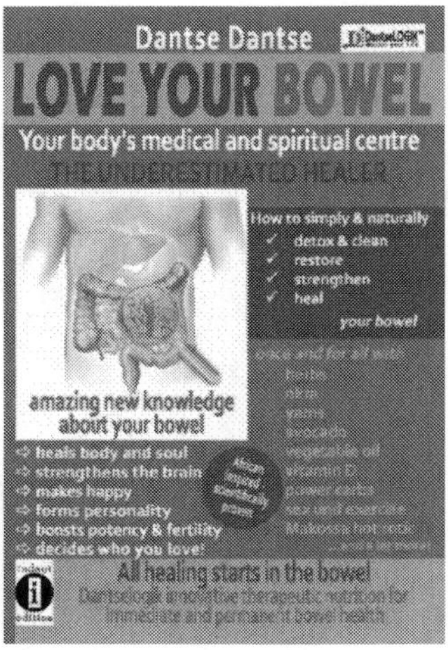
Dantse Dantse
LOVE YOUR BOWEL
Your body's medical and spiritual centre
THE UNDERESTIMATED HEALER
How to simply & naturally
detox & clean
restore
strengthen
heal
your bowel
amazing new knowledge about your bowel
heals body and soul
strengthens the brain
makes happy
forms personality
boosts potency & fertility
decides who you love!
All healing starts in the bowel
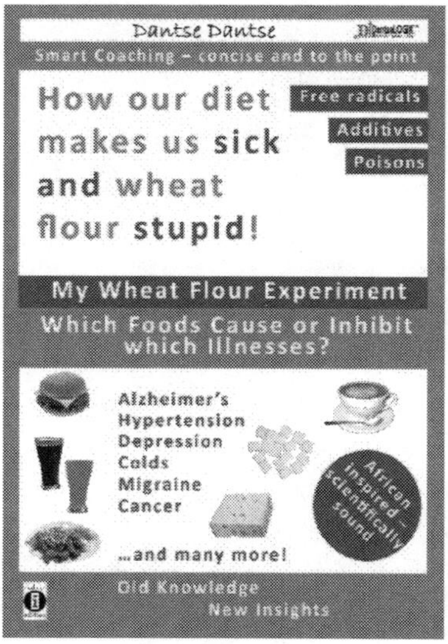
Dantse Dantse
Smart Coaching – concise and to the point
How our diet makes us sick and wheat flour stupid!
Free radicals
Additives
Poisons
My Wheat Flour Experiment
Which Foods Cause or Inhibit which Illnesses?
Alzheimer's
Hypertension
Depression
Colds
Migraine
Cancer
...and many more!
African inspired – scientifically sound
Old Knowledge
New Insights
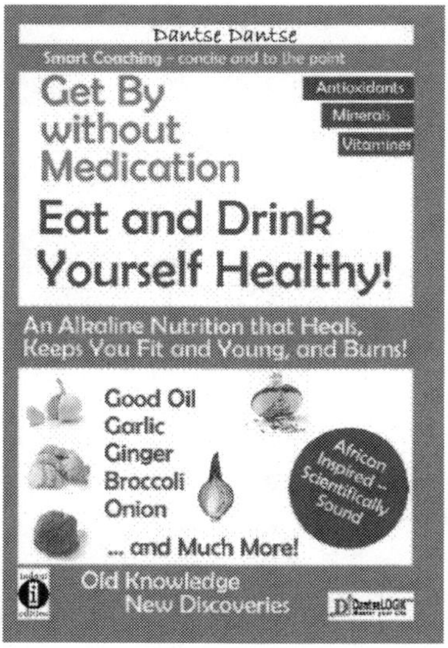
Dantse Dantse
Smart Coaching – concise and to the point
Get By without Medication
Antioxidants
Minerals
Vitamines
Eat and Drink Yourself Healthy!
An Alkaline Nutrition that Heals, Keeps You Fit and Young, and Burns!
Good Oil
Garlic
Ginger
Broccoli
Onion
... and Much More!
African Inspired – Scientifically Sound
Old Knowledge
New Discoveries

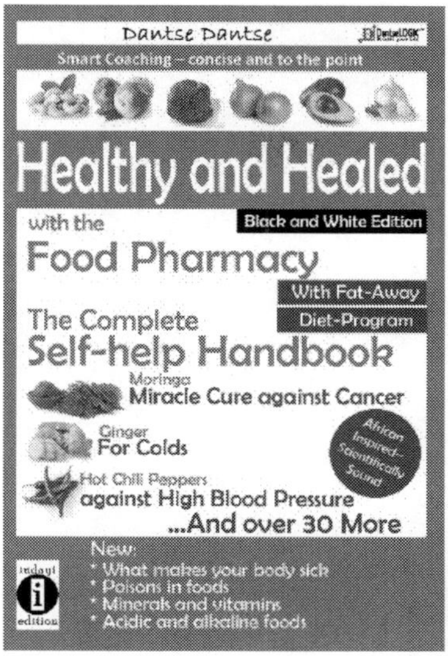
Dantse Dantse
Smart Coaching – concise and to the point
Healthy and Healed
with the
Black and White Edition
Food Pharmacy
With Fat-Away
Diet-Program
The Complete
Self-help Handbook
Moringa
Miracle Cure against Cancer
Ginger
For Colds
Hot Chili Peppers
against High Blood Pressure
...And over 30 More
New:
* What makes your body sick
* Poisons in foods
* Minerals and vitamins
* Acidic and alkaline foods

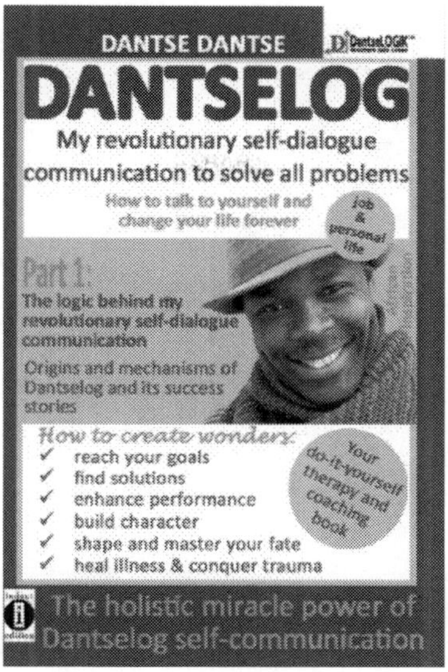
DANTSE DANTSE
DANTSELOG
My revolutionary self-dialogue
communication to solve all problems
How to talk to yourself and
change your life forever
Job & personal life
Part 1:
The logic behind my revolutionary self-dialogue communication
Origins and mechanisms of Dantselog and its success stories
How to create wonders:
✓ reach your goals
✓ find solutions
✓ enhance performance
✓ build character
✓ shape and master your fate
✓ heal illness & conquer trauma
Your do-it-yourself therapy and coaching book
The holistic miracle power of
Dantselog self-communication

Made in the USA
Coppell, TX
05 November 2026

11299176R00236